Instructor's Manual to Accompany Comer
ABNORMAL PSYCHOLOGY

Janet A. Simons, Ph.D.
Central Iowa Psychological Services

Ronald J. Comer, Ph.D.
Princeton University

W. H. Freeman and Company
New York

Revised printing

ISBN 0-7167-2299-2

Printed in the United States of America

2 3 4 5 6 7 8 9 0 VB 9 9 8 7 6 5 4 3 2

CONTENTS

Topic Overview:
I. Defining Psychological Abnormality

  A. Deviance
    1. different than the standard of appropriate and normal functioning
    2. violates social norms
    3. different from culture to culture

  B. Distress
    1. some believe it must cause distress in addition to being unusual
    2. although unusual aspects can bring enjoyment, some unusual behavior is clearly abnormal whether or not distress is experienced
    3. indeed, euphoria and unrealistic sense of well-being can be part of diagnosis

  C. Dysfunction
    1. abnormal behavior that interferes with daily living
    2. culture plays a role because it defines effective daily living
    3. some dysfunctions do not indicate psychological abnormality, e.g., sacrificing heros

  D. Difficulties in Defining Psychological Abnormality
    1. the definition is culturally relative and very selective and subjectively interpreted
    2. Thomas Szasz was a vocal critic of labeling mental illness and preferred the term "problems in living"

II. Past Views and Treatment

  A. Ancient Views and Treatments
    1. although 25% of people currently have mental disturbances, mental illness is not a new concept
    2. early beliefs about causes of mental illness included magic and bad spirits
    3. Stone Age persons used a crude operation called trephination, perhaps to release evil spirits
    4. early cultures who used writing (e.g., Egypt, China, Israel) all wrote about demonic causes of mental illness
    5. one early treatment was exorcism, various methods of coaxing evil spirits from the body

1

B. Greek and Roman Views and Treatments
   1. mental disorders were described and named, including melancholia, mania, dementia, and hysteria
   2. striking symptoms, such as delusions and hallucinations, were named and described
   3. Hippocrates viewed the cause as brain pathology attributed to imbalance of bodily fluids called humors
   4. well-known philosophers and physicians also believed in treating mental illness in ways similar to physical illness
   5. treatments in these civilizations included supportive atmospheres, music, massage, exercise, baths, sobriety, vegetarian diet, bleeding, and restraints

C. Europe in the Middle Ages: Demonology Returns
   1. collapse of Roman Empire also a collapse of scientific reasoning
   2. plagues, war, and urban uprisings also undermined science and increased belief in evil spirits
   3. tarantism and lycanthropy, forms of mass madness in which persons simultaneously shared the same symptoms, were viewed as caused by demonic possession
   4. clergy engaged in mild to severe forms of exorcism for treatment
   5. toward the end of this period, hospitals and the medical view began to reappear

D. The Renaissance and the Rise of Asylums
   1. Johann Weyer was the first medical practitioner to specialize in mental illness
   2. growing use of home care and pilgrimages to holy shrines
   3. some hospitals and monasteries were converted into asylums, which over time became filthy and degrading in their treatment of patients
   4. England's "Bedlam" and Vienna's "Lunatics' Tower" are two examples of deplorable conditions for mental patients during this period
   5. some treatments intended to help patients, such as Benjamin Rush's drawing of blood from patients, were based on wrong ideas and were cruel rather than therapeutic

E. The Nineteenth Century: Reform and Moral Treatment
   1. reform in this time period is attributable to individuals making dramatic changes
   2. Philippe Pinel and Jean-Baptiste Pussin led significant reforms in France
   3. William Tuke led humane changes in Europe
   4. Pinel and Tuke's methods became known as moral treatment
   5. moral treatment in the United States was first embraced by Benjamin Rush, who adopted this strategy over his earlier harsh methods
   6. Dorothea Dix campaigned for and succeeded in getting better mental hospitals in the United States
   7. the decline of moral treatment was due to money and staffing shortages and too few professionals, which led to lower recovery rates
   8. along with this, prejudice grew and people viewed the mentally ill as strange and dangerous
   9. moral treatment worked with many patients, but others needed medicines and counseling techniques that were not yet created

10. Clifford Beers wrote *A Mind That Found Itself*, which informed many people about hospital conditions and the experience of mental illness
11. the somatogenic perspective was advanced by Emil Kraepelin's classification system and by the discovery by Richard von Krafft-Ebing that untreated syphilis caused the mental illness of general paresis
12. early medical treatments included hydrotherapy, insulin coma shock, lobotomies, tonsillectomies, and teeth extraction
13. the roots of the psychogenic perspective are hypnotism and Freud's psychoanalysis

III. Current Trends

    A. New Treatments for the Severely Disturbed
        1. the importance of psychotropic medications that actually affect the brain and alleviate symptoms
        2. a policy of deinstitutionalization, which has dropped the number of hospitalized mental patients in the United States from 600,000 in 1955 to under 125,000 now
        3. new emphasis on community mental health

    B. New Treatment Settings for Less Severe Psychological Problems
        1. mostly outpatient care
        2. inclusion in more medical health insurance

    C. Today's Practitioners - psychiatrists, clinical psychologists, counseling psychologists, educational psychologists, psychiatric nurses, psychiatric social workers

    D. Emerging Perspectives
        1. decline in psychoanalytic therapy
        2. more numerous, often competing, types of counseling
        3. more effective biological treatments

    E. The Emphasis on Research

IV. Organization of the Text

Learning Objectives:
1. Define abnormal psychology and know the goals of this area of psychology.
2. List the general characteristics of abnormal patterns of psychological functioning.
3. Describe the early historical views of abnormal psychology, including those of Stone Age cultures and the Greek and Roman empires.
4. Know the popular view of mental illness during the Middle Ages and how this belief affected society.
5. Contrast the treatment of the mentally ill during the Renaissance and during the sixteenth century.
6. Discuss the improvements in the care of the mentally ill during the nineteenth century and specifically know the contributions of Philippe Pinel, William Tuke, Benjamin Rush, and Dorothea Dix in these reforms.
7. Describe how both the somatogenic perspective and the psychogenic perspective emerged in the late nineteenth century.

8. Explain the relationship between the development of psychotropic drugs and the policy of deinstitutionalization.
9. Distinguish among the different specialties of professionals who work with people who have psychological problems: psychiatrists, clinical psychologists, psychiatric social workers, counseling psychologists, educational psychologists, and psychiatric nurses.
10. Describe the major characteristics of current psychological perspectives: psychoanalytic, behavioral, cognitive, humanistic-existential, and sociocultural.

Instruction Suggestions:
1. *Class Discussion.* Use the people listed in Box 1-1 to generate a variety of discussion topics. You might ask students if they know of other persons whom they could add to the list (e.g., Jane Fonda, eating disorder; Pete Rose, compulsive gambling). Discuss the variety of outcomes for these individuals. For example, Patty Duke was successfully treated for her bipolar disorder but Freddie Prinze and Ernest Hemingway both committed suicide. Discuss how some of these individuals have written books about their problems (e.g., Patty Duke's *Call Me Anna* and Mark Vonnegut's *The Eden Express*). You can bring up a discussion of the stigma of mental illness by discussing Thomas Eagleton's withdrawal as a Vice Presidential candidate due to past treatment for depression.

2. *Class Discussion and Outside Assignment.* Have students find newspaper articles, magazine articles, talk show guests, television programs, and/or films that deal with mental illness issues. Have them explore the quality of the coverage, the use of accurate or inaccurate images, the assumptions made about mental illness, and the usefulness of coverage. You can adapt this into a written course assignment.

3. *Class Discussion and Outside Assignment.* Ask students to visit local bookstores or public libraries to look at self-help books (you might assign different problems to the students). Have them evaluate the quantity and the quality of such books. Ask them to bring in specific examples of books that seemed to be fairly useful. You can adapt this into a written course assignment.

4. *Class Project and Discussion.* Have students work in small groups of no more than six. Have them write a list of words used to label normal persons and a second list of words used to label abnormal persons. After several minutes, collate the lists of the small groups into one master list. You should find that there are more words listed under abnormal than under normal persons. Ask the class to explain the length differences. Ask them to evaluate the positive and negative aspects of the list. You may wish to point out the origin of some of the words used to label abnormal persons (e.g., "lunatic" is derived from the old belief that the moon influenced behavior, and "rocks in your head" is from a Middle Ages belief of the cause of abnormality and street-corner "surgeons" who would cut the stones out to simulate a cure).

4

5. *Classroom Demonstration.* Start and maintain a file of newspaper clippings that depict the various criteria of abnormality (e.g., distress, dysfunction, danger, deviance) that you can use each semester, both in this first chapter and then again for each appropriate diagnosis. Develop your file so that it includes both well-publicized cases and smaller local cases (you might wish to remove names of individuals involved).

6. *Class Discussion.* Introduce students to the idea that besides dysfunctional individuals, other units can be dysfunctional—families, workplaces, neighborhoods, cultures. You might ask if any students have worked in a dysfunctional workplace (i.e., a "crazy-making job"). If yes, you can get them to describe aspects that were dysfunctional (e.g., vindictive personnel, chaotic management, rules that kept changing, confusion, blaming, unethical practices).

7. *Mini-lecture.* **The Biblical Tradition**
The textbook covers the early Greek and Roman cultures, and you can add to the lecture material by introducing students to early Judeo-Christian views on mental illness. Here are some points you may wish to include in your lecture.
*Both the Old Testament and the New Testament refer to evil spirits as the cause of mental illness. For example, in the Old Testament, King Saul's evil spirits are soothed when David plays his harp. In the New Testament, Jesus coaxes the evil spirits from a man and transfers the spirits to swine.
*Judeo-Christian tradition also is the source of some people's belief that homosexuality is a mental illness. This is based on the interpretation of part of the book of Leviticus that lists several prohibitions (including not eating shellfish and not wearing man-made fibers) and on the words of St. Paul (who seems to suggest that celibacy is preferred to heterosexuality too). Opponents of this interpretation suggest that the Bible's guidelines are set according to the cultural need for high procreation rates rather than any other aspect. Our strong Judeo-Christian tradition is a major reason why homosexuality was considered a mental illness until 1974. Since that year, homosexuality has not been a diagnosed mental illness—the debate remains in church settings for whether homosexuality is an appropriate lifestyle or always a sin.
*Because this tradition viewed mental illness as a punishment from God, the early Jewish culture did not develop mental treatments as did the Greeks and Romans. To do so would have meant going against God's wishes.
*The Talmud, or Jewish holy writings, viewed epilepsy as a punishment from God. Cruel stereotypes of epileptics existed well into the twentieth century, with religious beliefs being one reason for poor understanding of epileptics.
*The Talmud also stated that people's abnormal and sinful sexual behaviors led to mental illness in oneself or the resulting offspring. The wrong sexual behaviors included having sex during a women's menstrual period or before she went through purification, sex before a kindled lamp (sex not in the dark), sex in front of a mirror, and sex on the floor. Belief that sex and mental illness are connected has a long and continuing history—into the 1930s, the medical profession thought that masturbation could cause mental illness (there was even a diagnosis of masturbatory insanity).
*The Bible was also cited as a reason for the torture, prosecution, and death of hundreds of mentally ill persons who were accused of being witches in the Middle

5

Ages. The Pope decreed harsh treatment of the accused witches because of a passage in Exodus that read "Suffer not a witch to live."

8. *Lecture Additions.* Under the Middle Ages material, you might want to add that the phrase "rocks in your head" originated in this time period. Quacks used to perform pseudo-surgery on city street corners. A person troubled by negative emotions or other symptoms of mental illness would hire the quack, who would make a minor incision on the head, an assistant would give the "surgeon" a few small stones, and the surgeon would act as if the stones were being taken from the head. The stones were seen as being the cause of the abnormal behavior and the patient was now "cured." This is an appropriate time to introduce students to the concept of the placebo effect. Ask them if this procedure might have sometimes worked because of the belief system of the patients. Along with the "ship of fools" topic of Box 1-2, you can add that "a slow boat to China" is an equivalent phrase.

9. *Class Discussion.* Have your students debate whether the demonology model exists today and in what forms. Does evil exist? The devil? Is there a role for exorcism or spiritual healing in psychotherapy? You may wish to review parts of Karl Menninger's *Whatever Became of Sin?* or Scott Peck's *People of the Lie* to be able to add to the class discussion. According to Peck, evil consists of denial and projection. Therefore, in some families, parents refuse to see their own limitations and faults and project these aspects onto their own children—giving their children serious problems. This pattern is what Peck views as the essence of evil. You can introduce students to some of the excellent examples in Peck's book and also have them discuss examples that they see in many realms— families, workplaces, churches, politics, and the world arena. An additional aspect of this discussion can be to discuss the concept of "accidie" (Maslow writes about this in *Toward a Psychology of Being*) or the sin of not doing all that we know we can do—so often "sin" is discussed only in terms of things that were done that should not have been done.

10. *Class Discussion.* The text points out that early asylums grew so fast and were so underfunded and understaffed that they became filthy, degrading human warehouses. It is important to tie this earlier poor treatment of the mentally ill to problems that exist today. Not nearly as many mentally ill persons are warehoused in large mental hospitals today due to the deinstitutionalization policy of the last four decades, and more well-trained professionals exist today, but many people still "fall through the cracks" and mental health care is still greatly underfunded both for care and for research. One result that you can discuss here is that a significant minority of the homeless in America need to be helped for serious mental illness yet they are not getting this help. Another aspect to bring up here is that in most states mentally ill persons are being housed in jails even though they have not committed a crime. In 1991, the National Association for the Mentally Ill (NAMI) did a series of articles and press releases about the numbers of mentally ill who are spending time in jail rather than in a treatment facility.

11. *Mini-lecture.* **Clifford Beers' Mental Illness**
You may wish to get a copy of Clifford Beers' *A Mind That Found Itself*, which was published in 1908. Share with your class some aspects of Beers' treatment and especially his description of mental illness. Here are a few aspects that you can use about his mental illness:

*Clifford Beers had a brother who died from epileptic seizures and part of Clifford's delusional system was that he became convinced that he was doomed to get epilepsy. When Beers had the flu, he became convinced it was the start of his epilepsy.

*While in college, Clifford Beers refused to recite in his classes because he believed that was the situation that would trigger his first epileptic seizure.

*When he falsely believed that he had severe epilepsy, he tried to kill himself by jumping out a window in his house. Instead, he broke his leg and was bedridden. While bedridden he developed a number of severe symptoms. He came to believe that his attempted suicide was a crime, and he was to be tried for attempted murder and would be hung. He believed that the people around him were detectives looking for evidence. For example, the food he ate would be taken as "confessions" of different crimes. If he ate burnt toast, he was confessing to arson. In addition, all food began to taste like it was full of blood. He soon stopped eating.

*He heard false voices, saw faces in the dark, and read handwriting on his bed sheets.

*He believed his nurses were detectives and his brother was an imposter— someone who looked like his brother but was someone else (Capgras syndrome).

*He misunderstood statements. When his brother tried to reassure him that "he'd soon be straightened out" (at a sanitarium), Clifford thought it meant he was going to be straightened out at the end of a hangman's rope.

12. *Classroom Activity.* If you have a fairly large class, data collected from students will be sufficiently revealing. Otherwise, you may want to either accumulate data over sections and semesters or enlist the cooperation of students in a large general psychology class. Have students anonymously answer the following questions (agree, disagree, don't know) and figure out the percentages. Compare the students' responses with those gathered in a Benefits Watch Survey commissioned by the National Association of Private Psychiatric Hospitals (1991).
1. I will never need mental health treatment.
2. I would not want my boss to know about my mental health treatment.
3. My family and friends would be supportive of my mental health treatment.
Answers in the original survey:
1. 15% - agree; 73% - disagree; 12% - don't know
2. 37% - agree; 57% - disagree; 6% - don't know
3. 95% - agree; 4% - disagree; 1% - don't know
The National Association for the Mentally Ill suggests that these findings indicate a shift away from the stigma of getting mental health treatment. 63% of American adults think that mental health benefits are an important part of insurance coverage.

13. *Classroom Demonstration.* Consider having a hypnotherapist speak to your class and conduct a demonstration with volunteering students. You could also put a self- hypnosis tape on reserve at the library and allow students to try it and evaluate the process.

14. *Classroom Demonstration.* Find examples of symptoms and treatments in other autobiographical materials and share at the start of the course or during discussion of appropriate mental disorders. For example, Frances Farmer's autobiography includes descriptions of hydrotherapy and insulin coma shock as well as generally poor mental hospital conditions. Sylvia Plath's autobiographical novel *The Bell Jar* includes a description of electroconvulsive therapy. Greenberg's autobiographical novel *I Never Promised You a Rose Garden* includes descriptions of schizophrenia and hospital treatment.

15. *Classroom Discussion.* Have students discuss how what is considered normal and abnormal is influenced by culture. Here are two examples of cultural differences:
A. Chinese restaurants may serve dishes made from the following meat sources: bear, snake, scorpion, dog, and rat.
B. Among Filipino peasants, a central cultural orientation is the egalitarian motive—a strong belief that all people should be equal. There is no drive to acquire things or to improve one's standard of living, and social approval is more important than material possessions. Guiding aspects include: (1) Pakiksama, the emphasis on good feelings among people rather than on personal achievement; (2) the desirability of just meeting one's needs and the avoidance of personal improvement (discouraged through teasing, threats, gossip); (3) a belief that "all have a right to live," and those not meeting daily needs are helped; (4) failure to succeed in these goals leads to feelings of embarrassment and inferiority called hiya.

Chapter 2. Models of Psychological Abnormality

Topic Overview:
I. The Biological Model

  A. Origins of the Biological Model
    1. Kraepelin's somatogenic theory
    2. research linking general paresis to syphilis
    3. effective psychotropic drugs in the 1950s

  B. Biological Explanations of Abnormal Behavior
    1. malfunctioning brain—either anatomically or biochemically
    2. organic mental disorders vs. functional mental disorders
    3. neural communication and neurotransmitters
    4. anxiety disorders linked to GABA, depression linked to low activity of norepinephrine and serotonin
    5. family-pedigree studies and risk studies explore mental disorders among biological relatives

  C. Assessing the Biological Model
    1. biological aspects of psychological processes
    2. research sometimes progresses rapidly
    3. some biological treatments offer significant help when other treatments have failed
    4. not always the appropriate model
    5. much research is inconclusive

II. The Psychodynamic Model

  A. Origins of the Psychodynamic Model
    1. Sigmund Freud studied hypnosis under Charcot and then worked with Breuer
    2. the case of Anna O. and the "talking cure" or "cathartic method"
    3. Freud's core of psychoanalysis is unconscious conflicts

  B. Freudian Explanations of Normal and Abnormal Functioning
    1. the id is one's instinctual needs, drives, and impulses, which uses reflexes and primary process thinking in accordance with the pleasure principle
    2. the ego seeks gratification in accordance with the reality principle via secondary process thinking
    3. the ego develops ego defense mechanisms to control unacceptable id impulses and to reduce the anxiety they arouse
    4. the superego is the value-laden aspect of personality that consists of the conscience and the ego ideal

5. in early childhood, individuals develop through psychosexual stages during which time they may become fixated, or entrapped, in development
6. the psychosexual stages are named: oral, anal, phallic, latency, and genital

C. Other Psychodynamic Explanations
1. Carl Jung focused on spiritual energy, the collective unconscious, and integrating opposing tendencies in the personality
2. Alfred Adler emphasized the drive to dominate others, feelings of inferiority, the inferiority complex, and the importance of social relationships
3. Erik Erikson emphasized lifelong development as a series of crises to resolve
4. Harry Stack Sullivan believed that emotional problems are caused by fear of human relationships
5. Karen Horney wrote that negligent or overprotective parents created "basic anxiety" in a child, which leads to strategies using helplessness, hostility, and isolation
6. Erich Fromm emphasized how people overcome isolation
7. Heinz Kohut divided the self into the core self, subjective self, and verbal self

D. Assessing the Psychodynamic Model
1. eloquent and comprehensive theories
2. abnormal functioning rooted in the same processes as normal functioning
3. poorly defined and hard to research
4. poor prediction of abnormal behavior
5. responsible for triggering the development of other therapeutic models

III. The Behavioral Model

A. Origins of the Behavioral Model
1. developed in psychological laboratories
2. applied to modifying abnormal behaviors since the 1920s

B. Classical Conditioning and Explanations of Abnormal Behavior
1. Pavlov's research
2. basic paradigm: UCS, UCR, CS, CR
3. the development of phobias or fetishes

C. Operant Conditioning Explanations of Abnormal Behavior
1. Thorndike and Skinner
2. law of reinforcement and shaping
3. drug use as reinforcing; schizophrenic symptoms as attention-getting

D. Modeling Explanations of Abnormal Behaviors
1. observation and imitation
2. imitation of aggressive behaviors

E. Assessing the Behavioral Model
1. can be tested in the laboratory
2. research models may not reflect real-life complexities
3. overemphasis on overt behaviors and underemphasis on cognitive behaviors

IV. The Cognitive Model

    A. Origins of the Cognitive Model
        1. in 1950s, social psychologists interested in attributions
        2. growing interest in cognitive behaviorism in the 1960s

    B. Cognitive Explanations
        1. maladaptive assumptions or basic irrational assumptions
        2. specific upsetting thoughts involving automatic thoughts and counterproductive self-statements
        3. illogical thinking processes, such as selective perception, overgeneralization, and magnification

    C. Assessing the Cognitive Model
        1. views human thought as a major contributor
        2. testable
        3. in some cases thoughts can be a consequence instead of a cause

V. The Humanistic-Existential Model

    A. Origins of the Humanistic-Existential Model
        1. Carl Rogers viewed clients as center of their own treatment
        2. Existentialists viewed individuals as in the process of being and developing uniqueness

    B. Humanistic Explanations of Abnormal Behavior
        1. unconditional positive regard versus conditions of worth
        2. constant self-deception makes it impossible for people to self-actualize

    C. Existential Explanations of Abnormal Behavior
        1. self-deception involves hiding from life's responsibilities
        2. failing to give meaning to life, thus not using one's capacity and freedom
        3. overreliance on authority and excessive conformity

    D. Assessing the Humanistic-Existential Model
        1. focuses on broad human issues
        2. optimistic tone
        3. difficult to research
        4. heterogeneity

VI. The Sociocultural Model

    A. Origins of the Sociocultural Model
        1. from sociology and anthropology
        2. societies generate abnormal behavior in their members
        3. mental illness and social class
        4. development of family theory and therapy in the 1950s

    B. Sociocultural Explanations of Abnormal Behavior
        1. family structure and communication, such as double-bind communications

2. societal stress, such as social change, social class, ethnic background, racial and sexual prejudice, and cultural institutions and values
3. societal labels and reactions, including the effects of having been labeled mentally ill
4. Rosenhan's study of pseudopatients in hospital settings

C. Assessing the Sociocultural Model
1. therapists more sensitive to the role of family and culture in the development of mental disorders
2. hard to get accurate research results from epidemiological studies
3. the most severe mental disorders tend to be universal rather than cultural
4. doesn't predict for individuals

VII. Relationships between the Models

A. Best to View Several Aspects Together than One Aspect at a Time

B. Different Kinds of Causal Factors
1. predisposing factors occur long before the disorder
2. precipitating factors trigger the disorder
3. maintaining factors keep the disorder going over time
4. diathesis-stress explanations propose a predisposition and an exposure to immediate stressors

Learning Objectives:
1. Be able to define paradigms or models and explain why they are useful in abnormal psychology.
2. Describe the main aspects of the biological model and evaluate its usefulness.
3. Describe the main aspects of the psychodynamic model and evaluate its usefulness.
4. Describe the main aspects of the behavioral model and evaluate its usefulness.
5. Describe the main aspects of the cognitive model and evaluate its usefulness.
6. Describe the main aspects of the humanistic-existential model and evaluate its usefulness.
7. Describe the main aspects of the sociocultural model and evaluate its usefulness.
8. Compare and contrast the various models for their assumptions and conclusions.
9. Explain the concept of diathesis-stress.

Instruction Suggestions:
1. *Classroom Activity*. List the different models (e.g., biological, psychodynamic, behavioral, cognitive, humanistic-existential, sociocultural) across the blackboard. Then ask students to list words, ideas, and names that they associate with each of the models. This activity is a good way to reintroduce students to the models and helps them realize how much they already know about the different paradigms. Of course, you can fill in some of the notable gaps. A real plus of this activity is that you can assess the knowledge of students near the beginning of the semester and use this information to provide lecture material at the needed level.

2. *Mini-lecture.* **The Brain Blood Barrier (bbb)**

You can make different perspectives "come alive" by featuring some current topic from the perspective. For the biological perspective, you might want to present material of the brain blood barrier. Both *Scientific American* and *Discover* magazine have recently done understandable and interesting articles on the bbb so you can brush up on the topic beforehand. Here are some ideas you can include in your lecture:

*The walls of blood vessels are different in the brain than in other parts of the body. As a result, fewer substances can get into the brain than can flow freely into other bodily organs.

*Usually this is a very good thing. For example, the bbb is effective in keeping the hallucinogen LSD out of the brain. Less than 1/10 of 1% gets into the brain. Can you imagine the results if even more got into the brain?

*However, some brain diseases are difficult to treat because the effectiveness of the bbb makes it hard to get needed medications into the brain itself. Scientists are developing ways to "trick" the bbb when needed.

*The capillaries in the brain make up only 5 percent of its volume but add up as 400 miles of vessels. The unique structure of these capillaries is that they have a continuous wall called the endothelium, and this endothelium is surrounded by astrocytes, one type of glial cells. The endothelium is composed of lipid molecules; as a result, water-soluble molecules (e.g., albumin, sodium, penicillin) cannot cross this wall easily, but lipid-soluble molecules (e.g., nicotine, ethanol, heroin, caffeine, valium, codeine) can cross the endothelium easily.

*One way to determine the addictiveness of illicit drugs is by how easily the substance passes through the bbb. Using this method, nicotine and cocaine are the two that pose the biggest problem. Both easily pass through the bbb and can quickly alter the brain. No wonder that cigarettes and crack are two difficult drugs to give up.

*Some non-lipid-soluble molecules that are essential to brain functioning (e.g., glucose, some amino acids) are transported across and others are synthesized by brain cells.

*The antiluminal membrane, or "metabolic" blood-brain barrier, is a second barrier. Some substances (e.g., L-dopa) can cross the endothelium but not the antiluminal.

*Heroin gets through the bbb more easily than does morphine. As a result, heroin is stronger and more addictive. Moreover, once heroin is in the brain, it changes back into morphine, making it difficult to pass through the antiluminal membrane and leave the brain—a double-whammy effect. Methadone gets through the bbb even more easily than heroin and thus is more addictive than heroin, yet it is used in treating heroin addicts because it does not give as pleasurable an experience as does heroin.

*Some medications can enter the brain readily because they are lipid-soluble (e.g., the antibiotic chloramphenolcol), but others are blocked from the brain because they are not lipid-soluble (e.g., penicillin). Researchers are looking for ways to get around this blockage so that more medications can treat brain infections. Possible solutions? Injecting the carotid with a hyperosmotic sugar solution (e.g., mannitol), which temporarily lowers the bbb (however, other unwanted substances can then also enter). Or, inject substances directly into the cerebrospinal fluid. Or, modify the substance to get it through the bbb and then have it alter again so that it does not come back out (much as heroin operates).

13

3. *Class Discussion.* Let students know that accurate genetic testing is now available for the genetic disorder of Huntington's disease. Family members can be tested before making reproductive decisions to know if they might pass this dominant gene disease on to offspring. All individuals with the genetic marker would develop this degenerative, fatal disease in middle age; those who tested free of the genetic marker would never get this disease. Without testing, a person with a parent with Huntington's disease has a 50% change of having the disease. Testing takes the odds to 100% or to 0%. If this disease was in your family, would you get the genetic test done and find out whether you (and potentially your offspring) were destined for the disease or cleared of the possibility? More have chosen not to get the test. Why?

4. *Class Demonstration.* Give your students this study aid developed by Don Irwin at Des Moines Area Community College to help them remember the neuron's parts: Have them look at their hand and think of the fingers as dendrites (a neuron can have several), the palm as the soma or cell body, and the thumb as the neuron's one axon. Tell them to visualize an impulse beginning at the fingers (dendrites), moving down their palm (soma) and down their thumb (axon), where it then communicates to their other hand's (neuron) fingers (dendrites).

5. *Mini-lecture.* **A Different Translation of Freud**
    You can use material from Bruno Bettelheim's *Freud and Man's Soul* to have students get a fresh view of Freud. The following are a few of Bettelheim's ideas:
        *Freud is poorly translated into English.
        *Freud chose the term psychoanalysis because it translated as "soul analysis," and Freud viewed therapy as a spiritual journey of self-discovery.
        *Freud can be interpreted as suggesting the need for a spontaneous sympathy of one's unconscious with that of others.
        *Libido, which is translated as sex drive, is better translated as sensual drive. Bettelheim says, "Although Freud is often quoted today in introductory psychology texts...his writings have only superficially influenced the work of the academic psychologists who quote him....American psychology has become all analysis—to the complete neglect of the psyche, or soul." (p. 19)
        *The child may fall in love with his parent, but the child also wishes not to be able to fulfill this desire or to harm the parent.
        *Destructive consequences occur from acting without knowing what one is doing.

6. *Classroom Discussion.* After describing the penis envy of Freud's Electra complex, you can introduce Karen Horney's concept of womb envy. Basically, Horney suggested that males envy the female ability to be pregnant and give birth and deal with this envy by belittling motherhood, pregnancy, childbirth, and feminine achievements. Have students evaluate the concepts of castration envy, penis envy, and womb envy. Do they have relevance in any or all cultures? It has been proposed that they are specific ways of expressing power envy. What do you students think about that idea?

7. *Classroom Project.* If you did not do a demonstration of hypnosis with Chapter One, you might want to assign a self-hypnosis project option in relationship to the origins of the psychodynamic model.

8. *Lecture Additions.* In your lectures, it is good to include several examples of interactions among the perspectives—both supportive and critical exchanges. You might want to include some biological research that provides tentative support for Freud's concept of the unconscious. You can find material in Milner's December 1986 article in *Psychology Today* or in Jonathan Winson's *Brain and Psyche: The Biology of the Unconscious.*
   *Benjamin Libbit's research indicates that sensory processing requires about half a second to reach consciousness, yet the subjective experience is that one is aware of the sensation as it is occurring.
   *Jonathan Winson suggests that this half-second is the neurophysical basis of repression.
   *Howard Sherrin measures subliminal perception processing with evoked potential (EP) recordings and has found more EP to subliminal "meaningful" stimuli than to "less meaningful" stimuli. Also, repressors, or individuals who typically keep unpleasant feelings from conscious awareness, exhibit fewer EP to meaningful stimuli than do others.

9. *Mini-lecture.* **Freud and Seduction Theory**
   You might want to address Freud's early idea of seduction theory in which he dealt with the problem of incest and suggested that it was a common experience. Proposed before the turn of the century, Freud suggested that many of his clients were dealing with the aftermath of early sexual abuse by a family member. Met with outrage from professional colleagues, Freud publicly rejected his theory and instead proposed the fantasy versions of parental seduction of Oedipus complex and Electra complex. Privately he may still have continued to believe in his original seduction theory. To develop a good lecture, become familiar with the writings of psychoanalyst Alice Miller, who has nicely addressed the effects of incest from a psychoanalytic framework. You can have the class discuss how society and treatment might be different if Freud had held to his original idea—would he have become an obscure theorist/doctor or would he still have become famous and been able to help earlier generations of incest victims?

10. *Lecture Additions.* A good addition to the section on classical conditioning is conditioned taste aversions. Students are interested in practical examples and you can give examples of taste aversions associated with chemotherapy and the flu. You can also relate Garcia's research on lithium-treated mutton and coyotes that then avoided sheep. Students may have some examples to provide.

11. *Class Activity.* An excellent way to introduce cognitive theory and the idea of irrational ideas and cognitive errors is to generate a list of common cognitive mistakes that college students make, such as "An A is the only grade worth earning" or "The teachers are out to fail us." You can use the following list from Freeman and DeWolf's *Woulda, Coulda, Shoulda* to aid students in developing relevant incorrect thinking examples.
   *All-or-nothing thinking, i.e., the world is all good or all bad, all gain or all loss
   *Catastrophizing, i.e., exaggerating the negative parts of an event
   *Comparing, i.e., judging by others rather than by one's own performance, feelings, and values

*Emotion reasoning, i.e., letting emotions overwhelm common sense
*Fortune-telling, i.e., being disappointed at oneself for not being able to predict the future
*Mind reading, i.e., jumping to conclusions about what others think or what they think you are thinking
*Overgeneralization, i.e., thinking that if something has happened once it will always happen
*Perfectionism, i.e., requiring oneself to perform flawlessly
*Unquestioning acceptance of critics, i.e., letting others define one's self-worth

12. *Class Discussion.* Using Erich Fromm's book *To Have or To Be*, introduce students to the idea of a having mode and a being mode. Have them discuss the difference in self-definition and self-evaluation based on one's possessions, property, and ability to take and get things versus self-definition and self-evaluation based on one's activity and being. How do values differ? Goals? Language? Mental health?

13. *Lecture Additions.* Tell students about Murray Bowen's ideas about family triangles and how they distort family situations and hinder solving family problems. In the wicked-stepparent triangle, there is open conflict between stepchildren and stepparent with the biological parent caught between the two sides trying to defend one or both sides. The perfect-stepparent triangle is when the stepparent is the rescuer who "straightens out" the child or "makes up" for the past. The ghost-of-the-former-spouse triangle is when marital parents end up in conflict over alimony, child support, and visitation issues. Finally, the grandparent triangle involves many forms of reactivity to former in-laws and is acted out by rules about grandparenting. In therapy, more realistic expectations for a stepfamily are encouraged and the real hurts and angers are identified and dealt with.

14. *Classroom Discussion.* When addressing the sociocultural explanations of abnormal behavior, point out factors that are associated with high rates of mental illness—such as poverty. Ask students what kinds of clients they would like to serve. Where would they like to practice (private practice or an inner city agency)? Introduce the concept of YAVIS clients—the kinds most professionals want to see. YAVIS clients are those that are young, attractive, verbal, intelligent, and social. In other words, clients that are (1) less needy than others, (2) have more resources to recover, (3) are the most like the professionals, and (4) who already have many options for getting better. What general societal biases are exhibited by the preference for YAVIS clients?

15. *Lecture Addition.* Expand upon Rosenhan's study called *On Being Sane in Insane Places* that is briefly covered in the text. You can mention that one of the pseudopatients was a professional artist and her work was interpreted by staff in terms of her illness and recovery. At one hospital, games donated by a women's club were kept locked up so that they would be new-looking if the club ever checked up on their condition. As the pseudopatients took notes about their experience, staff members referred to the note-taking as schizophrenic writing. In Rosenhan's writing on this study you can locate more interesting examples.

Chapter 3. Research in Abnormal Psychology

Topic Overview:

I. The Task of Clinical Researchers

    A. use scientific method
    B. search for general truths
    C. identify and explain relationships between variables

II. The Case Study

    A. Example: Freud's Little Hans case

    B. Value of the Case Study
        1. information that has implications for the person's treatment
        2. provide tentative support for a theoretical position
        3. challenge a theoretical position
        4. can study unusual problems

    C. Limitations of the Case Study
        1. biased observing—subjective and unsystematic
        2. low internal validity
        3. little basis for generalization

III. The Correlation Method

    A. Basic Characteristics
        1. look at "co-relationship" of variables
        2. process of operationalization
        3. representative sample of subjects

    B. The Direction of Correlation
        1. line of best fit
        2. positive correlation and negative correlation
        3. unrelated variables

    C. The Magnitude of Correlation
        1. strength of relationship
        2. accuracy of predictions

    D. The Correlation Coefficient
        1. +1.00 and -1.00 are perfect correlations
        2. zero correlation shows no relationship
        3. the closer r is to .00, the weaker the correlation

E. Statistical Analysis
    1. determining the real correlation in the general population from the
       sample of subjects
    2. statistically significant— probably not due to chance

F. Strengths and Limitations of the Correlational Method
    1. more external validity than case study but lacks internal validity
    2. describe and predict but not explain

G. Special Forms of Correlational Research
    1. epidemiological studies determine the incidence and prevalence of a disorder in a
       given population
    2. longitudinal studies look at the same subjects over a long period of time

IV. The Experimental Method

A. Basic Characteristics
    1. situation is manipulated and the effect is observed
    2. hypothesis is tested
    3. manipulated variable is independent variable and dependent variable is observed

B. Confounds
    1. major obstacles in isolating the true cause
    2. examples are confounds of time and situational variables

C. The Control Group
    1. group of subjects not exposed to the independent variable
    2. shows effects of passage of time and other confounds
    3. a comparison group for experimental group(s)

D. Random Assignment
    1. problems with self-selection
    2. greatly reduces chances of subject bias

E. Blind Design
    1. subject bias, such as trying to help the experimenter out
    2. placebo effects
    3. experimenter bias caused by subtle changes in experimenter behavior
    4. Rosenthal effect, after first psychologist to clarify the effects of experimenter bias
    5. double-blind studies

F. Statistical Analysis
    1. determine if differences are due to chance
    2. findings of statistical significance increase one's confidence that results are due to
       the independent variable

G. Variations in Experimental Design
    1. quasi-experimental design does not randomly assign subjects but uses groups that already exist
    2. natural experiments involve nature rather than experimenter manipulating the independent variable
    3. analogue experiments involve inducing subjects to behave in ways they believe to be like real-life abnormal behavior
    4. single-subject experiments involve using baseline data to compare treatment results on a single subject

Learning Objectives:
1. Discuss the problems that exist when doing clinical psychology research.
2. Describe the scientific method.
3. Describe the characteristics of the case study method.
4. List the advantages and disadvantages of the case study method.
5. Describe the correlation method and the statistical analysis involved.
6. Know the advantages and disadvantages involved with the correlational method.
7. Describe the experimental method.
8. Know how researchers reduce the effects of confounds by using control groups, random assignment, and blind designs.
9. Describe the variations of experimental designs that are used for ethical and practical reasons.

Instruction Suggestion:
1. *Class Discussion.* This chapter begins with the example of how clinical psychologists used to believe that schizophrenia was caused by schizophrenogenic mothers. This chapter beginning allows for a class discussion of how psychologists have often blamed mothers for causing mental illness (more than blaming fathers). Have students discuss their beliefs and attitudes about mother-produced mental illness. Some students might be familiar with Bly's *Iron John*, which proposes that father's time in the workplace resulted in boys winning the Oedipal complex with their mothers, which left them weak and emasculated. Psychoanalyst Melanie Klein proposed that paranoid personality was caused in infancy from having a mother with "stony breasts." Have them think of other examples in which moms get the blame. Do they agree?

2. *Lecture Additions.* The chapter defines nomothetic and idiographic truths. You may wish to discuss Gordon Allport's advocacy of the idiographic method as worthy of personality psychologists. You can describe his own work with "letters from Jenny."

3. *Classroom Demonstration.* Hand out to half the students the problem 1 x 2 x 3 x 4 x 5 x 6 x 7 x 8 and to the other half the problem 8 x 7 x 6 x 5 x 4 x 3 x 2 x 1. Have them guess the solution within 5 seconds of receiving the problem. (The correct answer is 40,320.) Students receiving the first problem will average lower guesses than those who receive the second problem.

Have half of the students answer the following: Given that there are 1,000 annual cases of electrocution, how many people do you think die from fireworks each year? Give the other half this question to answer: Given that there were 50,000 annual deaths from car accidents, how many people do you think die from fireworks each year? In one study, persons given the first question guessed 77 and those given the second question guessed 331. The actual answer was 6.

Hand out a list of 20 problems to solve. Ask half to indicate (before attempting the problems) whether they expect to get above or below 18 right and then to estimate the actual number that will be correct. Ask the rest to indicate whether they expect to get above or below 4 correct and to estimate the actual number. The first group will give a higher estimate. Research by Daniel Cervone suggests that if you actually allow students to work on the problems the first group will (1) try longer to solve the problems and (2) actually get more solved.

All of these dramatic problems demonstrate the effects of framing, a major type of thinking error. Amos Tversky and Daniel Kahneman also found that subjects are influenced by purely random numbers (the blasting effect of a seemingly random number) in that when subjects spun a wheel of numbers and then were asked to estimate the percentage of African countries in the United Nations, when the wheel said 10 they estimated an average of 25 percent but when the wheel was on 65 they estimated an average of 45 percent.

In one study, 829,000 high school seniors were asked to rate their ability to get along with others. Not one person gave a self-rating of below average; 60 percent ranked their abilities in the top 10 percent, and 25 percent ranked themselves in the top 1 percent. There is a strong tendency to rate oneself as "better-than-average." Also, most people use a false consensus effect and overestimate the number of people who agree with their views. Another strong bias is the self-serving bias, or the tendency to take credit for one's successes and to explain one's failures as externally caused. However, not all people share this bias; depressed persons are likely to blame themselves for failure and dismiss the successes as a matter of luck.

4. *Lecture Additions*. The chapter describes the case of Anna O. Tell students that the real Anna O. went on to "buck" the Orthodox Jewish system and establish a high quality girls' school. After "Anna's" death and when the Nazis overtook Europe, Hitler planned to change this girls' school into a whorehouse with the current students being the prostitutes. Instead, all of the students poisoned themselves to avoid this fate.

5. *Classroom Activity*. Bring into the classroom some actual studies involving epidemiological research and longitudinal research. Interesting epidemiological research is often covered in *New England Journal of Medicine*, as well as psychology and sociology journals. You can use either recent studies or you can bring in "classic materials." Have students in small groups find the interesting features in these journal articles. Besides journals, appropriate materials can be found in government publications, such as prevalence of mental disorders and prevalence of drug use among high school students.

6. *Class Project and Discussion*. If possible, have students collect newspaper articles based on correlational studies. With the students, go over the articles and decide if the journalist correctly interpreted the results of the studies or if correlational results were used to indicate causation. If time does not permit the gathering of current articles, discuss the following correlation found by George Snedecor, who was a statistician at Iowa State University many years ago. Snedecor found a .90+ correlation between the importation of bananas and the divorce rate. In other words, if one year had more bananas delivered into the country, then it had more divorces than the other year, too. If correlations mean cause-and-effect, then, do bananas cause divorces? Or, do divorcing people eat more bananas? (Of course, as the population increased, there were more divorces and more bananas consumed.)

7. *Classroom Activity*. Have students read actual (or made up) titles of research articles and point out which is the independent variable (IV) and which is the dependent variable (DV). Point out that one popular title form is The effects of (IV) on (IV).

8. *Mini-Lecture*. **The Rosenthal Effect**
The chapter mentions that experimenter bias is referred to as the Rosenthal effect. You can relate the initial classic work of Rosenthal to dramatically illustrate to students how experimenters bias studies. At the end of your presentation, you can expand the material into a class discussion of bias effects in the classroom and in the mental health arena.
   *Present material about how Rosenthal had graduate students teach rats to run mazes. Each rat was run an equal amount of time daily. Although rats came from the same litter, students were led to believe that they had either a rat genetically bred to be "maze bright" or genetically bred to be "maze dull." Although genetically similar, those rats whose trainer thought they were "maze bright" did perform better than the supposedly "maze dull" rats. It seems that rats who were expected to do better were subtly better encouraged than were the "dull" rats.
   *In a related study, the experimenter went into a slow-learners class and gave a pseudo-test that was designed to pick out "late bloomers," students who were currently behind their age norms but who had hidden potential. In actuality, "late bloomers" were randomly chosen and placed on a list. Near the beginning of a school year, teachers were briefly shown this list of "late bloomers" once. At the end of the year, these pseudo-"late bloomers" had actually outperformed the rest of the class. Perhaps the moral for teachers is to assume that every student has this hidden potential—and perhaps then it will appear.

9. *Class Discussion*. Have students discuss other natural experiments, such as survivors of the Holocaust and Vietnam Vets' PTSD.

10. *Lecture Additions*. When lecturing about the use of animals in research, you might mention that it was difficult to find laboratory animals that willingly would drink alcohol for research in that area. Rats and cats only learned to prefer their spiked water and spiked milk if under very stressful circumstances, such as receiving repeated electric shocks. At one time the gerbil seemed to be the perfect alcoholic animal— drinking lots of alcohol and getting "drunk" (as one researcher put it, "drinking until

they would lie stretched out on their exercise wheel"). However, gerbils did not stay as "hung over" as humans. After a few hours they were active and energetic. It seems that gerbils have livers that process alcohol much faster and more efficiently than do humans. Therefore, research with gerbils would not be very relevant to human alcohol effects. Among other solutions, rats that crave alcohol have been bred.

11. *Mini-Lecture.* **Early Views on Animal Research**
Your students may be aware of how some people are now protesting how animals are used in research. You might share some information about the Victorian antivivisectionist movement with your students. These ideas are found in a March 1990 *American Psychologist* article by Dewsbury.
    *Around the time that nineteenth century psychology was developing an experimental physiology that relied heavily on animal subjects, England and the United States were starting humane and antivivisection movements.
    *Henry Bergh founded the American Society for the Prevention of Cruelty to Animals on April 21, 1866.
    *William James, the founder of American psychology, sought a balance between the need for animal experimentation and ethical research. James wrote, "Vivisection, in other words, is a painful duty." Also, "...to taboo vivisection is then the same thing as to give up seeking after a knowledge of physiology."
    *John Dewey also viewed animal experimentation as a duty. In 1926 he wrote, "Scientific men are under definite obligation to experiment upon animals so far as that is the alternative to random and possible harmful experimentation upon human beings, and so far as such experimentation is a means of saving human life and of increasing human vigor and efficiency."
    *The author of the first North American comparative psychology text, John Bascom, favored restricting vivisection so that pain was reduced to the lowest possible amount and doing only important experiments and limiting repetitive experiments.
    *Ivan Pavlov justified his animal research with "the human mind has no other means of becoming acquainted with the laws of organic world except by experiments and observations on living animals." He added, "When I dissect and destroy a living animal, I hear within myself a bitter reproach that with rough and blundering hand I am crushing an incomparable artistic mechanism. But I endure in the interest of truth, for the benefit of humanity." Yet, antivivisectionists accused Pavlov of enjoying the destruction of animals.
    *John B. Watson, who did anesthetized surgery on white rats that included removal of eyes, eardrum destruction, and removal of olfactory bulbs, was called "killer of baby rats" in the media. One reporter wrote, "Now, if the same experiments were tried on the inspired Watson himself the results would be better, as he could tell us all about it. But he prefers to keep his eyes in his own head. So would the rats."
    *An important outcome of this early animal rights and antivivisection movement was that the American Psychological Association appointed a committee on animal experimentation in 1925 to establish research guidelines for animal studies. Today, the APA Committee on Animal Research and Ethics (CARE) sets standards for animal use in research, ensuring the continuance of humane animal research.

Topic Overview:
I. Clinical Assessment

    A. Uses
        1. determining how and why a person is behaving abnormally
        2. deciding appropriate course of treatment
        3. evaluating effectiveness of counseling
        4. conducting research
        5. using assessment techniques that are compatible with theoretical orientation

    B. Clinical Interviews
        1. conducted face-to-face
        2. the technique that instinctively seems the best
        3. almost always part of a clinical assessment
        4. conducting the interview involves establishing rapport and gathering data consistent with one's orientation
        5. can be structured or unstructured
        6. problems include that information is preselected by client, the information may be biased or inaccurate, subjective judgments are involved, and responses differ by interviewer qualities

    C. Clinical Tests
        1. useful tests are standardized and have reliability and validity
        2. the four kinds of reliability are test-retest reliability, alternate-form reliability, internal reliability, and interrater reliability
        3. the types of validity are face validity, predictive validity, concurrent validity, content validity, and construct validity

    D. Projective Tests
        1. projective tests include the Rorschach Test, the Thematic Apperception Test, sentence completion test, and drawings
        2. projective tests have not demonstrated high levels of reliability and validity and suffer from the absence of appropriate normative data

    E. Personality Inventories
        1. personality inventories include the Minnesota Multiphasic Personality Inventory, the Edwards Personal Preference Schedule, and the Q-sort
        2. inventories take less time to administer and score compared to projective tests and are more likely to have norms
        3. greater validity and reliability

F. Self-Report Inventories
   1. used to collect detailed information about one narrow area of functioning
   2. self-report inventories may assess emotions, social skills, thought patterns, or reinforcement patterns
   3. strong face validity and efficiency, but lack response-set scales and have not usually been standardized or assessed for reliability and validity

G. Psychophysiological Tests
   1. interest began when studies suggested that anxiety was accompanied by physiological changes
   2. often used in assessment and treatment of sexual disorders
   3. biofeedback used in assessing and treating medical problems, such as headaches and hypertension

H. Neuropsychological Tests
   1. neurological problems may be detected by CAT scans, EEG, PET scans, NMR, brain X rays, and brain surgery and biopsy
   2. subtle abnormalities may be revealed by neuropsychological tests, such as the Bender Visual-Motor Gestalt Test or the Halstead-Reitan Neuropsychology Battery

I. Intelligence Tests
   1. the most widely used intelligence tests are the Wechsler Adult Intelligence Scale, the Wechsler Intelligence Scale for Children, and the Stanford-Binet Intelligence Scale
   2. carefully constructed, large standardization samples, high reliability and validity, but scores can be affected by aspects that have little to do with intelligence and items can be culturally biased

J. Integrating Test Data
   1. using a battery of tests
   2. allows the strengths to be used and the weak points minimized
   3. adds information to the clinical interview

II. Clinical Observations

A. Naturalistic and Structured Observation
   1. clinician or a participant observer may conduct the naturalistic observation
   2. when naturalistic observation is impractical, can observe clients in a structured setting
   3. common problems include observer drift, observer bias, and subject reactivity
   4. clinical observations can lack cross-situational validity, or external validity

B. Self-monitoring
   1. subjects observe themselves and carefully record specific behaviors, feelings, or thoughts
   2. may record frequency or circumstances
   3. need for good instructions
   4. strong reactivity effect

III. Clinical Interpretation and Judgment

  A. Interpreting Assessment Data
     1. a sample of typical behavior
     2. correlates or predictive uses
     3. forming of hypotheses and testing them

  B. How Clinicians Test Hypotheses
     1. an additive, or linear model
     2. researching logic and biases used

IV. Diagnosis

  A. Classification Systems
     1. a syndrome is a cluster of symptoms
     2. guidelines for assigning to categories
     3. useful in describing, studying, and communicating
     4. Emil Kraepelin developed the first influential classification
     5. Kraepelin's system formed the foundation for the International Classification of
        Diseases (ICD)
     6. the ICD is in its tenth revision (ICD-10)
     7. the American Psychiatric Association developed the Diagnostic and Statistical
        Manual of Mental Disorders (DSM)

  B. DSM-III-R
     1. the DSM was revised in 1952 (DSM-I), 1968 (DSM-II), 1980 (DSM-III), and 1987
        (DSM-III-R)
     2. a DSM-IV is scheduled for publication in 1993
     3. the current form is more comprehensive than its predecessors
     4. diagnosis can be made on five axes, or information areas
     5. Axis I are vivid disorders that cause significant impairments
     6. Axis II are long-standing disorders that persist in fairly stable forms
     7. Axis III lists current physical ailments
     8. Axis IV lists severity of psychosocial stresses
     9. Axis V information is a rating of psychological, social, and occupational
        functioning currently and for the past year

  C. Reliability and Validity in Classification
     1. DSM-III-R is more reliable than predecessors because more objective criteria are
        provided
     2. etiological validity is shown by the similar backgrounds of individuals who have
        one diagnosis

  D. Problems of Clinical Misinterpretation
     1. clinician biases such as gender, age, race, socioeconomic
     2. too much weight given to first data
     3. overweigh one type of information
     4. "reading-in syndrome"

E. Dangers of Diagnosing and Labeling
   1. diagnostic labels may be self-fulfilling prophecies
   2. Rosenhan's study
   3. stigma attached to abnormality

Learning Objectives:
1. Describe the role of assessment, interpretation, and diagnosis in working with clients.
2. Know how psychodynamic clinicians use assessment differently than behavioral and cognitive clinicians.
3. Compare structured and unstructured clinical interviews.
4. Explain the reliability, validity, and standardization of clinical tests.
5. Compare and contrast the features of and uses for projective tests and personality inventories.
6. Describe psychophysiological tests.
7. Describe neuropsychological tests and know why they are used.
8. Know what intelligence tests do and what their shortcomings are.
9. Know about clinical observation and the three procedures of naturalistic observation, structured observation, and self-monitoring.
10. Know characteristics of a classification system and be familiar with the major features of the DSM-III-R.
11. Discuss the difficulties involved in making correct diagnoses.
12. Explain the harm that can be caused by the labeling process.

Instruction Suggestions:
1. *Classroom Demonstration.* Bring into your class available examples of personality inventories, projective tests, and intelligence tests and share a few aspects of the tests with your students. If possible, include a few of the tests mentioned in this chapter, e.g., MMPI, Rorschach Inkblot, TAT, WAIS-R, and so on. Have students give their reaction to the test content.

2. *Classroom Demonstration.* Bring a copy of the DSM-III-R to class and point out its features. Read one of the diagnostic criteria sections to the students. Ask them if it is similar to what they thought it would be.

3. *Class Activity.* Divide students into small groups and tell them they are supposed to view themselves as counselors. In this role, they are to develop a list of information that they would most want to know from a client at the end of the first session together. Then have the groups share their lists and develop one master list. Discuss what their impressions of important information are and why. Two variations are possible: (1) assign different counseling perspectives to the small groups and (2) assign a specific client type (e.g., schizophrenic, divorced male, battered woman).

4. *Class Activity.* Assign students different theoretical orientations and give them a client description. Have some students act out the client role and the other students interview the client from the assigned perspective. Psychoanalytic and behaviorist therapists make nice contrasts.

5. *Classroom Activity.* For each of the following kinds of validity, have students provide examples that they have experienced in college: face validity, predictive validity, content validity, construct validity. Can students provide examples for when proper validity standards were not met?

6. *Class Project.* Assign students to find appropriate pictures from magazines (*Life, Time, Newsweek,* for example) for developing a quick TAT-like test. In pairs, have them take turns in telling stories about the pictures and assessing primary themes. Have students express their opinion about the worth of such an approach.

7. *Class Activity.* Provide colored pencils or crayons and white paper to students and have them try one or more of the following drawing projective tests.
   A. Draw a mandala
   B. Draw a person, a house, and a tree
   C. Draw a picture of one's family
Have students write about or talk about one or more of their drawings. You can also provide information about how therapists use pictures such as these.

8. *Classroom Demonstration.* Locate and bring to class some older inventories and describe changes over the years (in older journals you might find questionnaires that measure neuroticism, for example; or you might look at Sheldon's inventories measuring ectomorphs, endomorphs, and mesomorphs).

9. *Classroom Demonstration.* Collect (or have students assemble) some questionnaires from popular magazines and/or self-help books. Compare these items with the more standardized, classic personality inventories, such as the MMPI.

10. *Class Discussion.* The MMPI mentions that one response set is social desirability. Bring in the items from the social desirability scale and read them to the class. Have them discuss why this response set occurs frequently.

11. *Class Project.* Have students develop and try out a Q-sort technique. One possible way to assign this is to have them come up with items that can be assessed as "True of the real me" and "True of my ideal me." Have students try their new test and evaluate what they learned from the activity in terms of test construction and in terms of self-knowledge.

12. *Classroom Demonstration.* Bring in and demonstrate biofeedback equipment (some inexpensive ones, including programs for computers, might be purchased by your psychology department). You can also use stress dot cards, which indicate level of stress by the color of the dot after being held ten seconds.

13. *Classroom Demonstration*. A growing area of assessment is neuropsychological testing. Demonstrate the Bender Visual-Motor Gestalt Test or the Halstead Reitan Neuropsychology Battery. Other simple tests can be found and adapted to the classroom.

14. *Classroom Demonstration*. Have a neurologist or a psychologist who does neuropsychological assessment come and speak to your class.

15. *Class Discussion*. Self-monitoring has the effect of helping to reduce a bad habit due to subject reactivity. In smoking, for example, writing a checkmark each time one lights up results in fewer cigarettes being smoked. This system can also be done by buying an expensive pocket computer to monitor (and later adjust) one's smoking habits. Do students think that the computer will produce better results than mere markings on a paper? Why, or why not? You can also discuss how to take other simple counseling ideas and use technology to develop a marketable product.

16. *Lecture Additions*. Under self-monitoring, you might want to address the differences between automatic and controlled processing. Habits are automatic, and therefore inflexible and hard to modify. Therapeutic intervention to change a habit is under controlled processing, which is changeable and flexible. One of the difficult aspects in long-term changing of habit is that the automatic processing can easily intervene. Controlled processing takes continual effort. So one person diets successfully for two weeks, keeping vigilant watch over fat content, number of calories, and so forth. Then, one slip-up, and the automatic processing leads to wiping out much of the constructive results.

17. *Classroom Demonstration and Discussion*. Bring in the DSM-I, DSM-II, and DSM-III along with the DSM-III-R. It is quite a dramatic visual impact to see how each version gets much longer. Have students discuss why DSM revisions gain in size.

Topic Overview:
I. Clients and Therapists

   A. Aspects Shared by All Therapies
      1. sufferer seeks relief from a healer
      2. healer is trained and socially sanctioned
      3. contacts are structured

   B. One-fifth of adults in the U. S. are in counseling

   C. A greater variety of problems are now being treated in counseling

   D. The most dominant counseling problems are anxiety and depression but 10 percent of clients have schizophrenia and 5 percent have substance abuse disorders

   E. Clients are no longer just the privileged, but a wide socioeconomic range

   F. Typically, clients wait an average of more than two years after the onset of symptoms before seeking counseling

   G. Length of counseling time varies, with more than half seeing counselors fewer than fifteen sessions

II. Systems of Therapy (employing a set of principles and techniques)

   A. Psychodynamic Therapies
      1. today's disorders result from previous emotional traumas
      2. insight therapy, i.e., uncovering old traumas
      3. main technique is free association
      4. interpretation especially of resistance, transference, and dreams
      5. catharsis, or emotional insight, is important
      6. shorter versions of psychodynamic therapies have been developed
      7. strongest support is from case studies, rather than systematic research

   B. Humanistic and Existential Therapies
      1. client-centered therapy emphasizes counselor qualities of unconditional positive regard, accurate empathy, and genuineness
      2. gestalt therapy involves skillful frustration, role-play, and exercises and games
      3. existential therapy encourages taking responsibility for one's life, freely making choices, and living an authentic life

C. Behavioral Therapies
   1. classical conditioning techniques include systematic desensitization and aversion therapy
   2. operant conditioning techniques include modifying behavior through rewards and punishments, and includes token economies
   3. modeling therapy is another type of behavioral therapy
   4. behavioral therapies have been shown to be effective for specific problems, such as reducing specific fears and social deficits

D. Cognitive Therapies
   1. rational emotive therapy uncovers irrational assumptions and challenges and modifies them
   2. cognitive therapy is most frequently used with depression
   3. cognitive-behavioral therapies view cognitions as responses that can be altered by systematic reward or punishment
   4. these strategies appeal to therapists of many persuasions and perform well in research studies

E. Biological Therapies
   1. effective psychotropic drugs have been around since the 1950s
   2. drug categories include antianxiety drugs (or minor tranquilizers), antidepressant drugs, antibipolar drugs (including lithium), and antipsychotic drugs (or neuroleptic drugs)
   3. electroconvulsive therapy (ECT) developed in the 1930s is widely used to treat depression, and the current form of bilateral ECT has fewer serious side effects while staying effective
   4. lobotomies were largely done in the 1940s and 1950s and today's psychosurgery is much more precise

III. Formats of Therapy

A. Individual Therapy
   1. first form of modern therapy
   2. number and length of sessions varies, as do techniques

B. Group Therapy
   1. grew in popularity after WWII and is viewed as efficient, time-saving, and relatively inexpensive
   2. often composed of a particular client population
   3. curative features include guidance, identification, group cohesiveness, universality, altruism, catharsis, and skill-building
   4. psychodrama involves role-playing techniques such as mirroring, role reversal, and magic shop
   5. self-help groups are groups in which people with similar problems help and support each other without direct leadership of professionals

C. Family Therapy
   1. family systems theory states that each family has its own implicit rules, relationship structure, and communication patterns
   2. structural family therapy focuses on family power structures

D. Marital Therapy
   1. marital therapy can incorporate any major therapy system
   2. behavioral marital therapy helps spouses identify and change problem behaviors
   3. intimacy in a couple can be reestablished using core symbols

IV. Is Treatment Effective?

   A. Generally Effective
      1. in 1952, Eysenck said no, but his research methods and interpretations have been criticized
      2. most recent studies find therapy to be helpful

   B. Effectiveness of Particular Therapies
      1. effectiveness for behavioral, cognitive, and biological therapies has been supported
      2. psychodynamic and client-centered therapies have received some support
      3. any therapy seems to be more beneficial than being in a control group

   C. Particular Therapies for Particular Disorders
      1. behavior therapies most effective for phobic disorders
      2. drug therapy most effective for schizophrenia
      3. cognitive-behavioral therapies very effective for sexual dysfunctions
      4. cognitive therapy and drug therapy successful for depression
      5. combined therapy approaches often superior to single approach

Learning Objectives:
1. Know what all forms of therapy have in common.
2. Compare and contrast the features and goals of global therapies and specific therapies.
3. Describe the procedures and techniques of psychodynamic therapies.
4. Know the primary characteristics of humanistic-existential therapies.
5. Compare and contrast client-centered therapy, gestalt therapy, and existential therapy.
6. Know the behavioral technique categories of classical conditioning, operant conditioning, and modeling.
7. Understand the premise of cognitive therapies and how cognitive therapies are conducted.
8. Know the three main kinds of biological therapy: drug therapy, electroconvulsive therapy, and psychosurgery.
9. Compare individual therapy and group therapy.
10. Describe family systems theory, family therapy and marital therapy.
11. Evaluate the effectiveness of therapy.

Instruction Suggestions:
1. *Class Activity.* Find recent surveys on people's attitudes toward therapy. You might locate this material in recent journal articles or the *APA Monitor*. You can also contact your local chapter of the National Association for the Mentally Ill (NAMI) for information concerning their reporting on changes in attitudes. In their newsletter in 1991 they featured information concerning the significantly more positive attitudes of the

American population toward others and oneself being in counseling. Have students formulate a simple opinion survey of attitudes toward therapy (incorporate some of the questions from surveys you discuss in class). Ask students in the class to anonymously answer the poll and keep the results over the years of the class.

2. *Mini-Lecture.* **Brief Therapies**

A growing style of counseling is the brief therapy format, which developed both due to professional belief that significant progress can be made on a specific problem and due to insurance policies that will only pay for a limited number of sessions (e.g., 3-8) for most concerns. Brief therapies tend to be problem-focused, action-oriented, and deal with a limited number of concerns. Many brief therapists incorporate behavioral techniques and cognitive techniques most heavily.

For example, the brief therapist may ask the client to deal with the most important concern in the client's life and to divulge only information that affects this concern. The therapist will ask about past and current personal strategies of the client dealing with the problem and how these approaches have worked. Then, the therapist and client will work together to propose a new behavioral approach and evaluate the results.

The brief therapist asks the client to address these questions:
(1) What is the significant problem with which you are dealing?
(2) What have you tried in dealing with this problem that has not worked?
(3) Are there incidents when these failed strategies have had positive results? And, if so, is there anything you can remember that was different during these times?
(4) What can be tried at a different level or with some modification?
(5) What could be tried that has not yet been tried?
(6) How can you think differently about this situation? Behave differently? Feel differently?

Brief therapy can be highly effective in working out specific life problems. However, research has also shown that long-term counseling continues to bring increasing benefits to the client.

3. *Class Activity.*
Gather books that deal with dream symbols and use these pictures and words to discuss dream analysis in your classes. You could also ask students (ahead of time) to anonymously write down a couple of dreams that they have had and have students do a "lay" interpretation of them. In this activity, point out the differences in how Sigmund Freud, Carl Jung, and Fritz Perls approached the analysis of dreams. Some classes can get into a lively discussion of the value of dream interpretation.

4. *Class Discussion.*
Have the class discuss their beliefs about whether or not symptom substitution occurs. Be ready to provide some examples if students just dismiss the possibility. For example, is there oral substitution when a smoker quits smoking cigarettes—does the ex-smoker start eating more or biting nails as an unconscious substitution? What other explanations are there?

5. *Class Activity.* You may use student volunteers to demonstrate the various gestalt techniques. Give them a specific situation to roleplay (e.g., anger at a father who abandoned the family, depression about death of a sibling, coming to terms with poor grades at college) so that no student is made to reveal sensitive aspects of their lives. Demonstrate the exaggeration game, the hot seat, and the empty chair.

6. *Lecture Additions.* Often psychology students are given very little coverage of existential psychology and are relatively uninformed about existential philosophy or existential literature. Consider sharing excerpts from the writings of existential psychologists, such as Rollo May's "A Man in a Cage" or from existential plays and literature, such as Sartre's *No Exit* or Camus' *The Plague.*

7. *Classroom Demonstration.* Here, or later in the anxiety chapter, consider spending some time demonstrating systematic desensitization. You can perhaps have the class develop a hierarchy for a college issue (speech class anxiety, mid-term examinations anxiety) and take them through the progressive relaxation training (stop short of the process of pairing the hierarchy and the relaxation; instead describe what the future steps would be).

8. *Lecture Additions.* You can provide a vivid example of a version of aversion therapy for quitting cigarette smoking. One technique is to put several smokers in a small, poorly ventilated room and to make them smoke continually for forty minutes. This procedure makes positive aspects of smoking become negative ones as there is no more sense of relaxation, but instead watery eyes, scratchy throats, smoke-filled atmosphere, and a sense of nausea. Cigarette butts are allowed to accumulate over four or five sessions, and any vomit is left until the end of a single session.

You can either lecture about or have the class discuss ethical issues (e.g., every participant should have a complete description of the treatment ahead of time and agree to the negative aspects), combining this technique with other counseling techniques (e.g., in addition to aversive conditioning, each participant pays $200 into a kitty, half of which is dispersed to all non-smokers at six months and the rest dispersed to remaining non-smokers at one year), and other versions of aversive conditioning for cigarette smokers (e.g., use of pictures of cancer patients, use of electrical shock).

9. *Class Discussion.* Put this quotation on the board:
    "Anything worth doing, is worth doing badly." - Oscar Wilde
Ask for student reactions to this quote. Most students will dislike it and criticize it. Then suggest that there are many things that they would have liked to try in life except that they tell themselves that "I don't have time to be good at it" or "It's too late to learn that well" or "I should have taken lessons as a kid." As adults we might tell ourselves "It's too late to go to college," or "Even though I would love to take an art class I'd probably only get a C." Each of us limits our lives of pleasure because we can't do the pleasurable activity well. If you're fifty, take piano lessons if you always wanted to learn, even though it's not going to play at Carnegie Hall. If you're really interested in chemistry, take that class, even though your ability might lead to a C and a small dent in

33

your grade point average. Go ahead and sing that hymn during the church service, even though your voice is not angelic. The real message of Wilde's quote is that it is okay to give yourself permission to try something at which you might fail. It's okay to work on something even if mediocre is the very best you could ever do on the task.

10. *Class Demonstration.* Bring in a copy of the *Physician's Desk Reference (PDR)* and share the side effects of a few psychoactive drugs with the class. You might want to choose a few selections ahead of time (e.g., meprobamate or Miltown, diazepam or Valium, fluoxetine hydrochloride or Prozac, chlorpromazine or Thorazine, and haloperidol or Haldol).

11. *Class Activity.* You may have students roleplay a psychodrama situation. Again, it is best to provide the student volunteers with a specific problem with which to work so that no student needs to reveal a true concern with the class. An alternative is to bring a therapist who specializes in psychodrama to the class to speak and do a demonstration.

12. *Class Demonstration.* Begin a collection of literature and information about self-help groups, especially those with local groups. You may wish to share a list of local groups with class members. If school counselors run groups or have information about groups in the community, let students know that this information is available.

13. *Class Activity.* On one blackboard write the phrases: PROFESSIONAL COUNSELING and SELF-HELP GROUPS. Have students generate a list of advantages and disadvantages for each of these formats. You may need to help this list grow by asking questions such as, "Which of these formats ensures confidentiality?"

Chapter 6. Anxiety Disorders

Topic Overview:
I. The Fear and Anxiety Response

    A. Basic Characteristics
        1. physical symptoms: faster breathing, tense muscles, rapid heart rate, and nausea
        2. inability to concentrate
        3. distorted world perceptions

    B. Autonomic Nervous System
        1. sympathetic nervous system as "flight-or-fight" system
        2. parasympathetic nervous system restores body to normal
        3. complementary systems

    C. Trait and State Anxiety
        1. trait anxiety is one's general level
        2. state anxiety is anxiety variations as affected by situations

II. Phobic Disorders and Generalized Anxiety Disorders

    A. Phobic Disorders
        1. phobia is persistent, unreasonable fear of specific object, activity, or situation
        2. typical coping is avoiding the object or situation and not thinking about the phobia
        3. differ by age or stage of life
        4. phobic disorders are more disruptive than phobias and are fairly common
        5. DSM-III-R distinguishes three categories: agoraphobia, social phobias, and simple phobias
        6. agoraphobia most pervasive and complex and leads to avoidance of public places and situations from which escape seems difficult should physical symptoms develop
        7. social phobias involve incapacitating exposure to scrutiny and may be specific or general
        8. majority are simple phobias, the persistent fear of objects such as thunderstorms, flying, and insects

    B. Generalized Anxiety Disorders
        1. in previous diagnostic systems called anxiety neurosis
        2. characterized by free-floating anxiety, or chronic and persistent anxiety
        3. 6% have symptoms and more common among women
        4. symptoms must be present at least six months and characterized by muscular tension, autonomic hyperactivity, and vigilance and scanning

5. may also exhibit mild depression or at another time be expressed as phobic disorder
6. pervasive anxiety is frustrating for family and friends as well as for the sufferer

C. Explanations of Phobic and Generalized Anxiety Disorders
  1. sociocultural explanation focuses on role of dangerous situations and societal pressures
  2. living near Three Mile Island nuclear power plant produced long-term elevated anxiety and depression levels
  3. cross-cultural studies indicate anxiety symptoms increase with a variety of societal changes, including war, political oppression, and modernization
  4. Freud distinguished three kinds of anxiety: realistic, neurotic, moral
  5. Freud thought people attempt to control unacceptable impulses by using ego defense mechanisms
  6. psychodynamic explanation of phobic disorders is that there is an overreliance on defense mechanisms, whereas generalized anxiety disorder is a breakdown of defense mechanisms
  7. phobias mostly involve defense mechanisms of repression and displacement
  8. Little Hans' fear of horses was interpreted by Freud as a displacement of castration anxiety
  9. defenses break down if poorly learned or under overwhelming stress
  10. some research findings consistent with psychodynamic explanation
  11. research findings could be explained differently, and not all findings are supportive
  12. Rogers believed anxiety disorders are caused by harsh self-standards, or conditions of worth
  13. existential anxiety is the fear of limits and responsibilities of existence
  14. anxiety disorders may be learned through conditioning
  15. fears can be classically conditioned or modeled and avoidance behaviors developed through operant conditioning
  16. animal and human research studies have supported behavioral explanations of anxiety disorders
  17. commonness of phobias may be determined by biological or cultural preparedness
  18. cognitive explanations center on maladaptive assumptions and faulty thinking processes
  19. unpredictability increases fear and generalized anxiety
  20. biological explanation first supported by effectiveness of benzodiazepines in treating anxiety
  21. generalized anxiety disorder is associated with the anxiety feedback system involving GABA and GABA receptors
  22. there are inborn differences in arousal styles
  23. generalized anxiety disorder runs in families and biological or environmental explanations can be offered

III. Panic Disorders

A. Panic Attacks
  1. panic attacks occur frequently, unpredictably, and without apparent cause
  2. they occur suddenly in harmless situations and last just minutes

3. symptoms: palpitations, tingling in hands or feet, shortness of breath, sweating, temperature changes, trembling, chest pains, choking sensations, faintness, dizziness, and a sense of unreality

B. Diagnosis of Panic Disorder
   1. four or more symptoms and four or more attacks within a month
   2. more common in young adulthood but no sex difference
   3. in previous diagnostic systems, seen as pattern of general anxiety
   4. a variation is panic disorder with agoraphobia, with agoraphobia emerging from the panic attacks

C. Biological Explanations
   1. in 1960s an antidepressant that affected norepinephrine shown to alleviate panic symptoms
   2. norepinephrine activity, especially in locus coeruleus, irregular in people with panic attacks
   3. yohimbine, which alters norepinephrine functioning, especially in the locus coerulus, can trigger panic symptoms even in those without history of panic
   4. blood pressure medicine clonidine affects norepinephrine and reduces panic symptoms

D. Cognitive-Biological Explanation
   1. panic-prone people are highly sensitive to physical sensations and overinterpreted them as signaling disaster
   2. worry about losing control, fear the worst, and lose perspective and end up with panic attack
   3. tendency to hyperventilate in stressful situations
   4. some have mitral valve prolapse (MVP), a cardiac malfunction marked by periodic heart palpitations

IV. Obsessive Compulsive Disorders

   A. General Information
      1. up to 2% suffer this disorder
      2. usually begins in adolescence or early adulthood
      3. no sex difference
      4. may also involve depression or alcohol abuse

   B. Obsessions
      1. feel both involuntary (ego dystonic) and foreign (ego alien)
      2. often as obsessive thoughts and wishes
      3. may be in form of repeated wishes or fantasies
      4. can involve images or ideas
      5. may involve the past or the future
      6. cross-culturally, dirt or contamination themes are most common, with other common themes being violence and aggression, orderliness, religion, and sexuality

C. Compulsions
    1. feeling compelled to do behaviors to prevent something terrible from happening while cognitively knowing the behavior is excessive and unreasonable
    2. compulsive rituals are detailed, elaborate performances of the compulsion
    3. common compulsion forms: cleaning compulsions, checking compulsions, symmetry, order, or balance compulsion, touching rituals, verbal compulsions, counting compulsions, and eating compulsions

D. Relationship between Obsessions and Compulsions
    1. 70% have both obsessions and compulsions
    2. compulsions often yielding to obsessive doubts, ideas, or urges
    3. less commonly, compulsions are used to control obsessions

E. Explanations of Obsessive Compulsive Disorders
    1. not well understood
    2. a battle between anxiety-provoking id impulses and anxiety-reducing defense mechanisms
    3. anal stage is especially important for development
    4. typical defense mechanisms are isolation, undoing, and reaction formation
    5. repetitive behaviors can develop through operant conditioning and are used to reduce anxiety levels
    6. serotonin and glucose metabolism may play important roles
    7. the antidepressant clomipramize may help reduce symptoms

V. Post-Traumatic Stress Disorder

A. Common Symptoms of PTSD
    1. reexperiencing the traumatic event
    2. avoidance
    3. reduced responsiveness
    4. increased arousal, anxiety, and guilt

B. Variety of Patterns
    1. any age
    2. mild to severe patterns
    3. soon after the traumatic event or a delayed onset

C. Post-Traumatic Stress Disorders Caused by Combat
    1. in previous wars called nostalgia, shell shock, and combat fatigue
    2. initially thought only 2% of Vietnam Vets suffered from PTSD
    3. more cases of delayed PTSD with Vietnam Vets
    4. 1/4 of 1.5 million Vietnam combat vets arrested within two years of return
    5. 200,000 dependent on drugs, higher divorce rate, higher suicide rate
    6. recollections triggered by similar stimuli, combat scenes, war news

D. Post-Traumatic Stress Disorders Caused by Other Traumas
    1. after natural and accidental disasters
    2. especially people who come close to dying or who lose family members
    3. survivors of Nazi concentration camps

4. rape trauma syndrome of high anxiety and startle responses, depression, guilt and self-blame, reliving the assault, nightmares, sleep disturbances

E. Explanations of Post-Traumatic Stress Disorder
1. greater risk if have other stressful life situations
2. less likely with strong support system
3. strong stressful situations will override positive personal and social context
4. prisoners of war often have PTSD despite previous good adjustment

VI. Anxiety Disorders: The State of the Field

A. Identifying Significant Differences in Various Anxiety Disorders

B. Phobic Disorders Best Understood and Obsessive Compulsive Disorders the Least

C. Contributions from Various Models of Psychopathology

D. Trend of Combining Viewpoints

Learning Objectives:
1. Distinguish between fear and anxiety.
2. List the five kinds of anxiety disorders and know their common components.
3. Explain the role of the sympathetic and parasympathetic nervous systems in the anxiety response.
4. Define phobia and describe the three kinds of phobic disorders: agoraphobia, simple phobia, and social phobia.
5. Describe the major features of generalized anxiety disorders.
6. Compare and contrast the various perspectives' explanations of phobic disorders and generalized anxiety disorders.
7. Describe the features of panic disorder and discuss the biological and cognitive-biological explanations of this disorder.
8. Distinguish between obsessions and compulsions.
9. Compare and contrast the psychodynamic, behavioral, and biological explanations for obsessive compulsive disorder.
10. Define post-traumatic stress disorder and list typical symptoms.

Instruction Suggestions:
1. *Class Demonstration.* Bring in the *DSM-III-R* and read one or more descriptions of various anxiety disorders. If you have access to the *DSM-II*, bring that into class and compare the current description of generalized anxiety disorder and the older version of anxiety neurosis. Elicit differences in the two or point them out. One significant difference to discuss is that the current manual is the first to suggest how long and how often symptoms should be present before using a specific diagnosis.

2. *Class Demonstration.* Get a copy of Charles Spielberger's *State-Trait Anxiety Inventory (STAI)*. Use this inventory to help you discuss the difference between trait anxiety and state anxiety. You might use college student examples to help illustrate these differences. For example, students can identify basic differences among college friends in their typical anxiety level; these differences represent trait anxiety. State anxiety can be

illustrated by having students draw a graph of experienced anxiety level across the semester. They will probably have a couple of "peak weeks" especially at mid-terms and finals. These differences illustrate the effects of state anxiety.

3. *Lecture Additions*. The text points out that "phobia" comes from the Greek word for fear. You can add that *Phobos* was the Greek god of fear. In fact, the scary face of Phobos was painted on the shields of Greek warriors to help strike fear into the hearts of their warring opponents.

4. *Lecture Additions*. The text mentions that many agoraphobics (and others with phobias) avoid driving in tunnels or on bridges. You might ask if any class members feel a little uneasy driving over high bridges. Those who do usually just experience a build-up in anxiety, get over the bridge, and then gradually relax. The question becomes then, what is experienced if the "bridge uneasy" person must travel across a very long bridge?

One such bridge crosses the Chesapeake Bay. This bridge is long enough to include a stopping area for a scenic view and roadside restrooms, and even some people who did not know that they were bridge phobic find themselves white-knuckled and paralyzed in fear along the side of the road. Authorities eventually solved some difficult problems by hiring experienced drivers to travel in vans until they noticed an incapacitated driver. They then would move the scared driver to a passenger seat and drive the car the rest of the way across the bridge.

5. *Class Activity*. Refer students to Box 6-1 and have them peruse the list of phobia names. Have students speculate on why phobias were given such "fancy names." Our favorite explanation is that when professionals can't treat and understand something we give it a name hard to pronounce so that the patient feels like progress is being made, and until behavior therapy techniques proved very successful, phobias were quite resistant to change. An interesting alternative, or addition, would be to select a few of these phobias and put them on flash cards. Choose words that some students will be able to figure out because of (1) familiar word root or (2) common words look similar and mean about the same. Have students figure out what these phobias represent. For example, you could choose the following phobias for this exercise:
    AEROPHOBIA (air) - aerogram, aeroplane, aero-
    APIPHOBIA (bees) - apiary
    PHOBOPHOBIA (fear) - phobia
    MONOPHOBIA (being alone) - mono-, monotone, monopoly
    ORNITHOPHOBIA (birds) - ornithology
    HEMATOPHOBIA (blood) - hematology
    BIBLIOPHOBIA (books) - bibliography, bibliotherapy, bibliophile
    CANCEROPHOBIA (cancer) - cancer
    ECCLESIAPHOBIA (churches) - ecclesiastic
    FRIGOPHOBIA (cold) - frigid, frigidaire
    CHROMATOPHOBIA (color) - trichromatic theory, kodachrome, chromatic
    CRYSTALLOPHOBIA (crystals) - crystals

DEMONOPHOBIA (devils) - demons, demonic
PHARMACOPHOBIA (drugs) - pharmacy, pharmaceutical
CHRONOPHOBIA (duration) - chrono-, chronicity, chronological, chronicle, chronic
ACROPHOBIA (heights) - acrobats, acropolis
CLAUSTROPHOBIA (enclosed space) - closets
ANGLOPHOBIA (England and English) - Anglosaxon, Anglo-American
ELECTROPHOBIA (electricity) - electric

6. *Class Activity.* Take a tally of phobias of class members (you can have them write them down to allow anonymity) and discuss the most common irrational fears. If the class is typical of the American population, public speaking will rank first (may be expressed as "speech class" among college students). It is also good to have class members determine which of the fears are simple phobias and which are social phobias. Sometimes this is easy (e.g., fear of storms, fear of spiders, and fear of bats are simple phobias), but sometimes social phobias might be mislabeled as simple phobias (e.g., fear of eating in restaurants and fear of blushing).

7. *Class Demonstration.* Ask a Vietnam Vet, a worker at a Vets Center, or a survivor of a natural catastrophe to speak to your class and discuss their experiences and what helped them to cope better.

8. *Class Discussion.* Propose some legal situations in which a victim of PTSD is involved and have the class discuss how PTSD affects how they would resolve the legal problem. Give a variety of situations and initial traumas—some that occurred over time and some that were an overwhelming, intense single event. For example, would a severely battered wife who has been physically and emotionally battered for seven years be considered a victim of PTSD? Why or why not? As jury members, would they consider this experience when considering the fate of a woman who shot and killed her husband during or after a battering?

Propose a situation in which a combat veteran has a flashback to a battle situation and assaults an ordinary citizen. Would you try the veteran? If you were on the jury, would it affect your decision? If convicted, what would be the best sentence?

You could also have small groups come up with a variety of legal situations and then discuss these class-generated situations as a whole.

9. *Lecture Additions.* Box 6-5 provides an interesting look at Howard Hughes' obsessive-compulsive behavior. You can add this additional information about his odd behavior:
   *Hughes would not touch any object unless he first picked up a tissue (which he called insulation) so that he would never directly touch an object that might expose him to germs.
   *Hughes saved his own urine in mason jars, storing hundreds of them in his apartment. From time to time a staff member would covertly empty some of the filled jars.

41

*Hughes saved his newspapers in high stacks, which sometimes led to visitors having to carefully weave through a room crowded with saved papers.
*Hughes sometimes watched one film (e.g., *Ice Station Zero*) more than a hundred times in a row before switching to another film. Likewise he might go for days eating the same couple of foods (e.g., chicken noodle soup and one flavor of Baskin-Robbins ice cream) and no others.
*Hughes used heroin and other drugs.

10. *Class Discussion*. Talk about dual-diagnosis and multiple-diagnosis. Individuals are not limited to just one diagnosis. After presenting the above additional information about Howard Hughes, you can have the class discuss for what diagnoses Hughes qualifies. Have students consider: obsessive compulsive behavior, agoraphobia, simple and social phobias, substance abuse, schizophrenia, paranoia, and personality disorders.

11. *Class Activity*. Have students generate a list of college situations that encourage anxiety symptoms and "mini" solutions that mimic phobias, obsessions, compulsions, free-floating anxiety, and so on. For example, are better term papers written if one finds a "healthy adaptation" of some of the obsessive compulsive qualities?

Topic Overview:

I. Global Therapies: Psychodynamic and Humanistic Approaches

    A. Psychodynamic Therapies
        1. anxiety disorders due to fear of id impulses and unsuccessfully controlling them
        2. get clients to uncover and understand unconscious issues
        3. somewhat helpful for generalized anxiety disorder but not the others
        4. free association and interpretation may increase obsessive compulsive pattern

    B. Humanistic and Existential Therapies
        1. therapeutic conditions: unconditional positive regard, empathy, genuine acceptance and concern
        2. help completely trust themselves and be more open and honest
        3. research not supportive of its effectiveness

II. Specific Therapies: Behavioral, Cognitive, and Biological Approaches

    A. Simple Phobias
        1. Wolpe's systematic desensitization involves learning to relax while confronted with feared objects or situations
        2. three phases of systematic desensitization: relaxation training, construction of fear hierarchy, graded pairing of feared objects and relaxation responses
        3. in flooding and implosive therapy, clients stop fearing things because of repeated, intensive exposure with feared objects, learning they are actually harmless
        4. modeling, or vicarious conditioning, involves therapist confronting the feared object or situation while client observes, with greatest effectiveness in participant modeling
        5. research supports behavioral approaches for simple phobias

    B. Agoraphobia
        1. a variety of in vivo exposure approaches
        2. support group approach involves agoraphobics going together into several-hour exposure situations
        3. another approach is home-based self-help programs
        4. about 2/3 of agoraphobics with exposure-based treatment are significantly helped
        5. exposure-based treatment less helpful for those with agoraphobia with panic disorder

C. Social Phobias
   1. one step is to reduce social fears by behavioral or cognitive therapy
   2. Ellis's rational-emotional therapy involves finding and altering irrational assumptions and doing homework assignments
   3. social skills training combines role-play, assertiveness training, and learning skills of social interaction
   4. results are best when cognitive therapy and social skills training are combined

D. Generalized Anxiety Disorders
   1. neither global nor specific approaches more than modestly helpful
   2. rational-emotive therapists identify and change anxiety-causing irrational assumptions
   3. Beck suggests their assumptions are dominated by themes of imminent danger
   4. working with automatic thoughts
   5. teach stress management skills to apply during stressful times
   6. stress inoculation to be able to replace negative self-statements with coping self-statements
   7. relaxation training and biofeedback are of modest help
   8. first medications were sedative-hypnotic drugs (e.g., barbiturates), which led to physical dependence, drowsiness, and overdose risk
   9. meprobamates (e.g., Miltown) were less dangerous but still caused drowsiness
   10. category of benzodiazepines (e.g., chlordiazepoxide and diazepam or Valium) reduced anxiety and were relatively nontoxic except when used with other drugs
   11. GABA receptor sites receive benzodiazepine drugs
   12. family physicians prescribe more benzodiazepines than psychiatrists do

E. Panic Disorders
   1. global therapies and stress management techniques not helpful
   2. antianxiety drugs do not reduce frequency or intensity of attacks
   3. antidepressant drugs prevented or lessened panic attacks
   4. alpraxolam (Xanax) is one benzodiazepine drug that is effective in treating panic attacks
   5. antidepressant drugs restore norepinephrine activity in the locus coeruleus
   6. antidepressant drugs and alprazolam help with panic disorder with agoraphobia
   7. misinterpretation of physical symptoms becomes a self-fulfilling prophecy leading to a panic attack
   8. taught to distract self from physical sensations

F. Obsessive Compulsive Disorders
   1. Frankl's paradoxical intention involved a direct, humorous confrontation of clients' thoughts, fears, and behaviors
   2. prevention of compulsion acts can lead to a reduction
   3. can repeatedly expose one to objects or situations that elicit obsessive fears but get client to refrain from compulsive act
   4. thought stopping, or saying "stop" to interrupt obsessive thoughts may lead to an intensification of obsessive thoughts
   5. antianxiety drugs not useful
   6. antidepressants, especially clomipramine, is helpful
   7. trichotillomania is helped with clomipramine

G. Post-Traumatic Stress Disorders
    1. treatment goals: reduce or overcome lingering symptoms, gain perspective on the trauma,and return to constructive living
    2. use of antianxiety drugs and antidepressant drugs to reduce tension, lessen nightmares, and reduce depression
    3. use of exposure-based techniques
    4. through talking and writing develop insight and perspective, bring out deep-seated feelings, accept experiences, become less judgmental of oneself, and learn to trust again
    5. group therapy to deal with guilt, overresponsibility, rage, and grief

III. Treatments for Anxiety Disorders: The State of the Field

    A. Many Changes Over Past 15 Years

    B. Behavioral and Drug Therapies Dominate Picture

    C. Cognitive Therapy Growing in Importance

    D. Better Matching of Patients with Treatment

    E. Research Helps Clarify and Alter Treatment

Learning Objectives:
1. Know how psychodynamic therapists explain anxiety disorders and what procedure they use.
2. Describe the three exposure-based behavioral therapies used in treating phobias: desensitization, flooding, and modeling.
3. Describe treatment for agoraphobia.
4. Know the two components of social phobias and how these components are treated using cognitive therapy and social skills training.
5. Explain why generalized anxiety disorders are least responsive to treatment.
6. List and describe the cognitive approaches, stress management training techniques, and benzodiazepine drugs used with generalized anxiety disorders.
7. Know how biological and cognitive interventions help in treating panic disorders.
8. Define paradoxical intention and in vivo exposure with response prevention and relate how they are used to help individuals with obsessive compulsive disorders.
9. Know what drugs are helpful for obsessive compulsive disorders.
10. Describe treatment programs for post-traumatic stress disorder.

Instruction Suggestions:
1. *Class Project.* Assign students to do (and record) a ten-minute attempt at free association. Have them begin with the thought, "One of the things I remember about the experience of anxiety is that...". Tell them to write about the experience of free association and to estimate their success at talking without censorship. At this point they should listen to their ten-minute session to refresh what they did think about. Then they should write about the cognitive flow during the free association. Did they change topics? Did some surprising topics come up? What are their reactions to their chain of associations?

Finally, they should state their opinions about the usefulness of free association in therapy. Would they like to enter therapy in which they were requested to engage in free association?

2. *Class Activity.* As a class or in small groups, have students construct a hierarchy of fears for a situation (other than one in the chapter). For example, a hierarchy to deal with (1) job interviews; (2) mid-term exams; (3) giving speeches in class. You may wish to instruct students in a muscle tension-relaxation exercise. Finally, describe the third step of pairing these two aspects together but do not do this step during class.

3. *Class Activity.* After emphasizing how vivid and detailed a description a therapist needs to be used with someone undergoing germ phobia and obsession, assign each small group the task of writing a graphic passage for one of the following examples. As groups work on this, check on their progress and suggest they need to add more vivid and disgusting detail (e.g., "Don't forget to describe the green mold that is growing on the slimy tomato left on that dirty dish in that filthy dish water," "Don't forget to describe those huge, mangy, flea-bitten, dirt-caked rats that run in and out of all that disgusting, smelling, leaking garbage at the dump"). At the end, dramatic read the small group passages, commenting that in actual flooding and implosive therapy more would be used for a greater length of time. Get class reactions to how these passages made them feel and what hearing a couple of hours of the passages would do.
   A. A sink full of dirty dishes that have gathered over a two-week period.
   B. A look into one of the most disgusting and filled garbage cans imaginable.
   C. A kitchen floor that has been unscrubbed for at least the last three months.
   D. Walking around a community junkyard.
   E. Taking a tour in a garbage dump.
   F. Viewing an underground sewer system.
   G. Looking into the refrigerator vegetable crisper after returning from a two-week vacation.

4. *Lecture Additions.* Here is a brief additional case of agoraphobia. Polly developed agoraphobia around the age of twenty when at home with two small children. Eventually, she could not shop in the back of the grocery store for fear that she would faint. She would not allow non-family members in her car because of her belief that it would trigger a panic attack. She did not go to concert halls, restaurants, or other public places because she believed her physical symptoms would develop and result in a loss of control. Malls especially were intolerable to her and she gave up the shopping sprees she had enjoyed as a teenager. In reality, Polly had only ever fainted twice.

Polly developed ingenious ways to cope with her agoraphobia. She had her best friend choose groceries located in the back of the store. She had her friends come to her home more than going to other homes and became quite a skilled hostess, cook, and entertainer. Friends were important to her and she honed her skills as a storyteller so that her agoraphobia did not leave her lonely. She did most of her shopping through catalogs.

Yet, Polly realized she needed help when her seven-year-old daughter needed new gym shoes and she sent Molly into the mall alone with a credit card to buy shoes. Molly succeeded and Polly thought that she needed to learn to be as courageous as Molly.

After a variety of therapy techniques that gradually expanded her world, the therapist had built Polly's self-esteem to the level that she tried college. However, she enrolled in a chemistry course because "I'd show my therapist that I wasn't smart enough for college and be done with this hard work of getting better" and enrolled in a night class "so if I fainted not as many people would see me embarrass myself." Polly never did faint and she managed a B in that first chemistry class. A year and a half later Polly had her A.A. degree, just over a year later she had a B.A. in psychology, and within two more years an M.A. in counseling.

5. *Class Activity.* Use "fear of blushing" to get students to design a combined cognitive therapy and social skills training program for a client.

6. *Class Demonstration.* Bring in a copy of the *Physician's Desk Reference (PDR)* and look up the information on some of the medications mentioned in this chapter and discuss the material in class.

7. *Class Activity.* Have the class generate typical automatic thoughts used by students, such as talking to oneself during a test with "you'll never finish," "stupid jerk," "everybody else can do this." Discuss the origin of the unhelpful automatic thoughts and how to reduce their power on us.

8. *Class Activity.* Discuss the material on stress inoculation and have students adapt this training for learning to cope better with mid-term exams (or some other threatening aspect of the semester). The four aspects are (1) Preparing for a Stressor (e.g., How many tests do I have? Which of them are comprehensive? What kinds of questions will be asked? How are the different tests schedule? What's my realistic plan of attack? Remember that I need to focus on what I *can* do to prepare for them); (2) Confronting and Handling a Stressor (e.g., I need to turn this stress into studying energy. Relax and be in control—remember to take deep breaths while studying and during the test.); (3) Coping with the Feeling of Being Overwhelmed (e.g., It's normal to feel scared while the tests are being past out—just let the feeling subside; I don't have to eliminate all my test anxiety—just keep it manageable); (4) Reinforcing Self-Statements (Way to go, you aren't dying! Hey, I recognize this one—see, you have learned a lot!).

9. *Class Demonstration.* Demonstrate biofeedback or stress cards in class. If you have stress dots, get students to wear them for one day and note what situations record as most stressful and most relaxed.

10. *Class Demonstration.* Ask a pharmacist, chemical dependency counselor, or physician to speak to your class about prescription drug addictions and the dangers of overdosing with prescribed drugs and over-the-counter medications.

11. *Class Discussion.* Have the class discuss how paradoxical intention might be applied to learning to cope better with one aspect of being a student.

12. *Class Demonstration.* Have a speaker from a Vets Center or other crisis center address the role of group therapy in dealing with PTSD.

13. *Class Project.* Have students keep a worry journal for a two-week period. At the end of that time period, either discuss in class or have them write a two- or three-page reaction to the experience of writing about their daily fears and anxieties.

Chapter 8. Mood Disorders

Topic Overview:

I. Unipolar Patterns of Depression

    A. Normal Dejection
        1. experienced by all of us
        2. seldom so severe that it significantly alters daily functioning
        3. beneficial if healthy self-exploration occurs

    B. The Prevalence of Unipolar Depression
        1. 6% of United States population, or 10 million persons, currently depressed
        2. worldwide, about 15% experience a severe episode sometime
        3. twice as many women have severe unipolar depression and also have more mild episodes
        4. no gender difference in depression between girls and boys
        5. any age, but especially men in their 50's and women from 35 to 45
        6. increasing incidence among teenagers and young adults
        7. 2/3 recover within 6 months but higher risk for reoccurrence

    C. Clinical Picture of Depression
        1. emotional symptoms include intense sadness, dejection, feeling empty, experiencing little pleasure, loss of humor, crying spells, and sometimes anxiety and anger
        2. loss of motivation to participate in one's usual activities, loss of drive and initiative, a "paralysis of will"
        3. between 7 and 15% commit suicide compared to 1% of nondepressed people—half of all suicides
        4. dramatic decrease in activity level, doing less and getting less done, moving slowing, lacking energy
        5. view self negatively and concluding one is inadequate, undesirable, inferior, unattractive, and perhaps evil
        6. blame themselves for nearly every negative event and rarely credit themselves for positive achievements, thereby being self-critical and full of guilt
        7. negative view of the future, not expecting things to improve, feeling hopeless
        8. complain that their intellectual ability, memory, and problem-solving abilities are deteriorating
        9. in problem solving, depressed do as well as nondepressed but predict poorer performances and evaluate themselves less favorably
       10. research found that depressed persons are less able to remember events of the distant past
       11. accompanied by physical complaints such as headaches, indigestion, constipation, dizziness, and pain
       12. disturbances in appetite and sleep are common, as is feeling tired

D. Diagnosing Unipolar Patterns of Depression
   1. a major depressive episode is severely disabling, lasts at least two weeks and has at least five symptoms
   2. if not the first episode, diagnosis is major depression, recurrent; first episode is major depression, single episode
   3. chronic depression indicates length over two years
   4. seasonal depressions fluctuate with seasonal changes
   5. melancholic indicates unaffected by pleasurable events, motor, sleep, and appetite disturbances significant, and very responsive to drug therapy
   6. less disabling depression and fewer than five symptoms is dysthymia for at least two years
   7. dysthymia leading to major depression is called double depression
   8. DSM-III-R dropped category of psychotic depression, but if psychotic features are present the diagnostician can indicate this

E. Recent Life Events and Unipolar Depression
   1. depressed persons tend to have experienced a greater number of stressful life events just prior to the episode
   2. those who have had stressful lives are more likely to become depressed as stresses multiply
   3. although external events can bring on unipolar patterns, the majority of depressed persons do not fit this pattern
   4. reactive depression indicates precipitating events and endogenous depression indicates internal causes
   5. today, unipolar depression is viewed as an interaction of internal and situational components

F. Explanations of Unipolar Patterns of Depression
   1. Freud and Abraham compared depression and grief
   2. not accepting grief leads to regression to oral stage
   3. introjecting the loved one leads to experiencing all their feelings toward the loved one as feelings about themselves
   4. as grief reaction worsens, feel empty, avoid relationships, become preoccupied with the sense of loss, and also experience self-hatred due to anger at a loved one for departing
   5. more prone if parents didn't meet needs of oral stage or if overgratified them
   6. if depressed without actual loss of loved one, Freud thought it due to imagined or symbolic loss
   7. vary in importance placed on the idea of hostility turned inward
   8. studies confirm that maternal separations up to the age of six years often accompany depression, a pattern called anaclitic depression
   9. Harlow's studies of separation and isolation in young monkeys showed a protest-despair reaction
   10. losing a parent before age five is associated with higher depression rates
   11. dreams of depressed persons have higher levels of hostility and masochism
   12. Lewinsohn proposes that depression is related to decrease in rewards and lower performance of positive behaviors
   13. a high rate of punishing experiences may also lead to depression
   14. when reinforcement rate rises, depressed persons improve
   15. social reinforcements are particularly important

16. reverse may happen—depressed mood changes behaviors and then reinforcement rate
17. Beck suggests that negative thinking (e.g., maladaptive attitudes, cognitive triad, errors in thinking, automatic thoughts) lies at the heart of unipolar depression
18. cognitive triad involves negative views about one's experiences, oneself, and the future
19. five common errors in logic are arbitrary inference, selective abstraction, overgeneralization, magnification and minimization, and personalization
20. the cognitive triad is typically experienced in automatic thinking
21. Beck's cognitive theory has received good support from research
22. Seligman suggests that helplessness is at the center of depression, including a perceived loss of control over reinforcements and yet holding oneself responsible for the helplessness
23. reverse helplessness by attributing losses of control to external causes or to internal causes that are specific or unstable
24. support for the genetic view comes primarily from family pedigree studies, twin studies, and adoption studies
25. the catecholamine theory looks at norepinephrine's role in depression
26. the idoleamine theory looks at serotonin's role in depression
27. current theories propose one or both of norepinephrine and serotonin as producing depression; others suggest acetylcholine

II. Bipolar Disorders

  A. Clinical Picture of Mania
    1. manic episodes involve out-of-proportion euphoric joy and well-being, activity, and expansive emotions but also irritability, anger, and annoyance
    2. motivationally, manic people want constant excitement, involvement, and companionship
    3. behavior of those with mania can be described as hyperactive, loud, fast, and flamboyant
    4. cognitively, manic persons display poor judgement and planning
    5. manic persons are energetic and get very little sleep, yet are wide awake

  B. Diagnosing Bipolar Disorders
    1. according to DSM-III-R, a manic episode is a predominantly elevated, expansive, or irritable mood and at least three other symptoms
    2. assigned bipolar disorder even if the depressed episode has not yet been experienced
    3. specific labels are: bipolar disorder, mixed; bipolar disorder, depressed; and bipolar disorder, manic
    4. milder manic episodes, or hypomania, leads to a diagnosis of cyclothymia

  C. Explanations of Bipolar Disorders
    1. psychodynamic view is that manic reactions are the denial of the loss of a loved one
    2. some believe oversupply of norepinephrine is related to mania
    3. like depression, mania is associated with a low level of serotonin
    4. another possibility is a neural imbalance of sodium ions

5. possible genetic predisposition to develop the biological abnormalities underlying bipolar disorders
6. genetic linkage studies, such as those done with Israeli, Belgians, Italian, and Amish families, help to identify possible patterns in the inheritance of bipolar disorders

III. Mood Disorders: The State of the Field

    A. Much Information Is Known about Mood Disorders Yet Not Yet Understood

    B. Unipolar Depressions Are Prevalent and Subside Eventually Even Without Treatment

    C. Bipolar Disorders Are Less Common but Patient Unlikely to Recover without Treatment

    D. Many Good Explanations for Unipolar Disorder but Only Biological Explanation Is Useful with Bipolar Disorder

    E. One Depression Symptom Capable of Affecting Others

Learning Objectives:
1. Be able to differentiate between moods and mood disorders.
2. Contrast unipolar depression and bipolar disorder.
3. Know the primary symptoms of depression and the relationship between depression and suicide.
4. Explain why women experience more depression than men.
5. Compare and contrast reactive depression and endogenous depression.
6. Describe the psychodynamic view of depression.
7. Describe the behavioral view of depression.
8. Define the four cognitive processes that generate depression symptoms: maladaptive attitudes, cognitive triad, errors in thinking, and automatic thoughts.
9. Explain the learned helplessness theory of unipolar depression.
10. Differentiate among internal-external, global-specific, and stable-unstable attributional dimensions.
11. Describe the possible roles of neurotransmitters and inherited predispositions in unipolar depression.
12. Define mania and describe the typical symptoms.
13. Describe bipolar disorder and know who is typically affected.
14. Distinguish between bipolar disorder and cyclothymia.
15. Know how biological research explains bipolar disorder.

Instruction Suggestions:
1. *Class Activity.* Have a class discussion on why depression is so common. List reasons on the blackboard. Then have students choose which of the items on the list are most common in the lives of college students. Are there additional reasons that they would give that pertain mostly to college students?

2. *Small Group Discussion.* Have students in groups of 3 to 6 share some of their own personal experiences with the five different areas of depression symptoms: emotional, motivational, behavioral, cognitive, and somatic.

3. *Class Activity.* Have the class help you develop a study aid that will help distinguish the various types of major depression and dysthymia (visual imagery is one possible tool).

4. *Lecture Additions.* Talk about the effects of anniversary reactions on depression. Explain how people may remourn a significant loss around the same time of year each year. If we lose a loved one around Christmas, Christmas customs can from then on be touched with sadness. Similar weather may also retrigger the emotion. It seems that the body may mourn even if cognitively one does not at first recognize the original loss. If one is depressed "just out of the blue" it might be a good idea to think about what losses occurred at "this time of year." Reacknowledging the losses and conducting a grieving ritual will help to reduce the length and intensity of the sadness. The losses are often people, but they may also be career changes, significant property losses, and major disappointments. Anniversary reactions are also associated with commencement of schizophrenic episodes.

5. *Lecture Additions.* While discussing the psychodynamic view that depression involves hostility turned against oneself, you might want to mention Karl Menninger's book *Man Against Himself*, which views all risk-taking behaviors as "a touch of suicide." Moreover, you might want to describe the Menninger Foundation and the Menninger Clinic in Topeka, Kansas, an institution that is the psychiatric version of the Mayo Clinic. Incidentally, if your college is within a few hours drive of Menninger, consider making arrangements to take psychology majors (or Psi Beta or Psi Chi members) to an arranged visit to the Menninger Clinic. Students will learn much from the tour.

6. *Mini-Lecture.* **The Monkey Studies of Harry and Margaret Harlow**
How does one choose as one's research subjects monkeys instead of rats or people? What significant event shapes the future research of a beginning psychologist? In Harry Harlow's case, his research path began when his graduate assistantship involved taking care of the monkeys in his college's Primate Laboratory. This unglamorous job included cleaning monkey cages. It seems that the infant monkeys had a soft diaper in their cages to use as a bed; therefore, Harlow had to launder lots of very dirty diapers. He noticed that the interval between taking the dirty diapers out and a couple of hours later when he put a clean diaper into each cage was spent with infant monkeys rocking themselves back and forth. Harry Harlow wondered just how important it was for young monkeys to have contact with something soft. This observation led to a lifelong series of studies by Harry and Margaret Harlow.

Harlow's most cited work is the one in which he found that monkeys preferred a cloth-covered surrogate mother monkey to a wire surrogate mother monkey that held a bottle. Harlow proposed that contact comfort was more basic than oral satisfaction.

The Harlow monkey studies of separation and isolation cited in this chapter are also well-known and were instrumental in furthering our knowledge about the protest-despair reaction. The Harlows also paired some shy, isolated monkeys with outgoing, social monkeys who played the role of "peer therapist." He then monitored the healthier responses of the young isolates. Another study involved forcing male monkeys to be "househusbands." In the wild, male monkeys are notoriously poor fathers, but the Harlows designed a cage that made male adult monkeys stay "home," and under these conditions the male monkeys became "better dads."

The Harlows contributed a wealth of knowledge to psychology, but it is important to avoid anthropomorphism when making scientific conclusions.

7. *Class Activity.* Bring in crayons (or colored pencils, waterpaints, fingerpaints, colored chalks) and large sheets of paper and have students draw a picture that represents depression and one that represents mania. You can have each student show their two pictures and explain them. Or, you could have them lightly write D or M on the back, shuffle the pictures, and see if the class can correctly put them into the two proper categories. Have them discuss if that was an easy task, and by what aspects they judged the pictures. You could assign this as an outside project and not limit the materials that are used.

8. *Small Group Discussion.* Assign one of the orientations (e.g., psychodynamic, behavioral, cognitive) to each group and have members come up with five suggestions to help a mildly depressed friend that fit the assigned orientation. Share results with the whole class.

9. *Class Project.* Ask each student to watch one episode of network news, one of local news, and to read the front page of a newspaper. Each student, to the best of his or her ability, is to rate each news item as either negative or positive. For each of the three assignments, tally all numbers given by students. Is the news more negative or more positive? Is any category more negative or more positive than the others? Why? In large classes you can compare the numbers for ABC, CBS, CNN, and NBC. Discuss the effects of news media on one's personal moods.

10. *Class Activity.* As you discuss the five common errors of thinking listed in the chapter (arbitrary inference, selective abstraction, overgeneralization, magnification and minimization, and personalization), list them on the blackboard, leaving room to write in examples. Have class members give examples of each type of thinking error that is common among college students. For example, magnification and minimization are shown by "Oh, well, anybody could have gotten an A in that easy class" and "I'll never succeed in a career now that I've gotten a C in that course." Have the class discuss the effects of thinking errors on their emotional state as a student. You might direct the discussion into ways to modify these common errors.

11. *Lecture Additions.* You might add into your lecture on cognitive theory and depression examples of maladaptive automatic thoughts that you have noticed students doing— like subvocally uttering "stupid jerk" to themselves when they see a C grade on a test. The student doesn't even realize the comment was made but feels down because of it. It also represents magnification in thinking since a C indicates average rather than failing.

12. *Class Demonstration.* Bring in a copy of Beck's Depression Inventory, or some other inventory about depression, and share some of the items of the inventory. Discuss the usefulness of these inventories in both therapy and research.

13. *Small Group Discussion.* Have students analyze and discuss the effects of learned helplessness and perceived lack of control in the lives of (1) college students; (2) children in foster homes; (3) terminally ill patients; (4) workers at a plant that is closing down; (5) political hostages. Try assigning a different person's situation to each group and then compare each group's list of effects. Are the groups' lists similar? Why or why not?

14. *Small Group Activity.* Have each small group design a situation that would lead to an increase in learned helplessness and therefore depression. Have them describe their situation to the other groups. What are the common elements? How do they differ?

15. *Class Demonstration.* Have a pharmacist come to your class and talk about the effects of psychoactive drugs on depression. Also, discuss how other medications (e.g., hypertension medicines) can lead to increased depression. Ask the speaker to evaluate the effectiveness of current medications, the advantages and disadvantages of drug therapy versus psychotherapy, and expectations about future medications.

16. *Lecture Additions.* Choose a literature selection(s) that depicts both depression and manic states and read it to the class. Sylvia Plath's *The Bell Jar* provides good examples.

17. *Class Demonstration.* Bring to your class a copy of the *Physician's Desk Reference (PDR)* and look up and share given side effects for lithium, tricyclics, and MAO inhibitors.

18. *Class Project.* Have students fill out a tally form for their favored explanation for gender differences in the incidence of depression. Rank each from first through fifth choice. In large classes, tally separately for females and males. In tallying the votes, add up the number of first place voices for each explanation. Eliminate the least popular option, and add the 2nd place choices of this option to the vote. In each round eliminate the least popular and go in turn to the alternative 3rd, 4th, and 5th place choices. At the end, you will have the choice that is most the most popular option.

You can also print out a form such as the one offered here and have students survey other students (anonymously).

	1st	2nd	3rd	4th	5th
1. Artifact hypothesis - Depression is underdiagnosed in men.					
2. X-linkage hypothesis- Since depression is a dominant mutation on the X chromosome, women run a higher risk.					
3. Traditional psychoanalytic explanation- Lifelong penis envy and vulnerability due to dependence on relationships to maintain self-esteem.					
4. Sociocultural explanation- Devalued housewives and overburdened working wives are prone to depression.					
5. Learned helplessness explanation- Vulnerability due to feeling little control over one's life.					

Topic Overview:
I. Treatments for Unipolar Patterns of Depression

  A. Psychodynamic Therapy
     1. grief over real or imagined losses must be brought to consciousness, understood, and resolved
     2. use free association to aid recall and therapist interpretation of associations, dreams, resistance, and transference
     3. therapist may take a more active role early in therapy than is typical
     4. extra care needed for the transference behaviors due to extreme dependencies
     5. goals: less dependent on others, more effective coping with losses, changes in daily living
     6. initial passivity and fatigue makes therapy more difficult, as does discouragement and leaving counseling prematurely

  B. Behavioral Therapy
     1. start with identifying reinforcing activities and introducing more of these
     2. in contingency management approach, systematic ignoring of the depressive behavior and rewards to constructive statements and behavior
     3. teach or reteach social skills
     4. group technique of personal effectiveness training in which members rehearse social roles, especially expressive behaviors
     5. combining Lewinsohn's behavioral techniques can be effective with mild or moderate depression

  C. Interpersonal Psychotherapy
     1. regardless of cause, Klerman and Weissman emphasize that all depression occurs in an interpersonal context
     2. if grief reaction involved, think about the loss and explore the lost relationship, including one's anger toward the departed person, then help in filling "the empty space"
     3. depression caused by interpersonal role disputes, or two people with different expectations about the relationship, leading to opening conflicts or hidden resentments and therefore depression
     4. some experiencing interpersonal role transition due to significant life changes
     5. another contributing cause is interpersonal deficits
     6. can be effective for mild to severe cases of unipolar depression

  D. Cognitive Therapy
     1. first phase is to increase activities and elevate mood
     2. second phase is to examine and invalidate automatic thoughts
     3. third phase is to identify distorted thinking and negative biases

4. fourth phase is altering primary attitudes
5. significant improvement has been demonstrated for mild to severe depressions

E. Electroconvulsive Therapy
   1. one of the most controversial forms of treatment for depression
   2. one of the most effective and fastest-acting interventions for severe unipolar depression
   3. unilateral ECT has largely replaced bilateral ECT and is much safer and as effective
   4. electrical current causes a convulsion of a few minutes' duration
   5. typically, 6 treatments are administered over two weeks
   6. in the 1930s von Meduna and then Cerletti worked toward the discovery of ECT
   7. Cerletti was the first to administer ECT to humans, used it for quite a while, and then abandoned it because of the side effects
   8. in early years, fractures, dislocations, and other problems fairly common
   9. today, muscle relaxants and barbiturates reduce both physical and mental trauma associated with this procedure
   10. the procedure is now more complex but less dangerous and less frightening
   11. unilateral ECT has reduced the danger of brain impairment
   12. ECT increases neurotransmitter activity in the brain
   13. decline in usage since the 1950s due to its history of abuse and the available alternatives in medications

F. Antidepressant Drugs
   1. before 1950s, only amphetamines were used to treat depression and they increased activity without alleviating the depression
   2. first MAO inhibitor affecting depression, iproniazid, was discovered accidentally while treating tubercular patients, however it caused serious liver damage
   3. better medicines (e.g., phenelzine, isocarboxazid, tranylcypromine, or Nardil, Marplan, and Parnate respectively) are MAO inhibitors that are used to stop the destruction of norepinephrine and serotonin
   4. the problem is that the enzyme MAO is essential for certain normal body functions, such as controlling high blood pressure
   5. if taking MAO inhibitors, MAO production in the liver and intestine are blocked, and tyramine can accumulate, so one must restrict diets of tyramine-containing foods
   6. tricyclic antidepressants (e.g., imipramine, amitriptyline, nortriptyline, doxepin, or Trofranil, Elavil, Aventryl, and Sinequan respectively) are effective with unipolar patterns and more commonly used than MAO inhibitors
   7. tricyclics alleviate depression by acting on reuptake mechanisms
   8. tricyclic side effects include tiredness, dry mouth, dizziness, blurred vision
   9. less dangerous and more effective than MAO inhibitors
   10. MAO inhibitors most effective with depression with symptoms of overeating, oversleeping, intense anxiety
   11. tricyclics most effective when major symptoms are slowed down, loss of appetite, insomnia
   12. second-generation antidepressants (e.g., maprotiline, amoxapine, trazondone, fluoxetine) do not inhibit MAO or affect reuptake process
   13. ECT more effective than antidepressant drug therapy

14. ECT especially considered with high suicide risk

G. Trends in Treatment
   1. unipolar depression can be effectively treated with cognitive, interpersonal, behavioral, and biological therapy
   2. most effective are cognitive, interpersonal, and biological therapies
   3. drug therapy reduces depression symptoms faster than cognitive and interpersonal therapies, but are matched by end of treatment
   4. behavioral therapy useful but not as effective
   5. psychodynamic therapies least effective
   6. combining cognitive therapy or IPT with drug therapy is most helpful

II. Treatments for Bipolar Disorders

A. Lithium Therapy
   1. lithium is a mineral salt that has greatly improved treatment for bipolar disorders
   2. correct dosage involves blood and urine analyses
   3. if unresponsive to or unable to tolerate lithium, carbamaxepine (Tegretol), an anti-convulsive drug, may help
   4. in 1949, Cade hypothesized that manic behavior is caused by a toxic level of uric acid and injected guinea pigs with uric acid made soluble with lithium, which instead made the animals lethargic, so Cade researched lithium
   5. lithium not approved for treatment until 1970 and since then research has supported its effectiveness in treating manic episodes
   6. a prophylactic drug because it helps prevent symptoms from developing
   7. also alleviates depressive episodes of bipolar disorders
   8. "second messengers" that alter synaptic activity in neurons using norepinephrine and serotonin by activating sodium ions
   9. lithium ions can substitute for sodium ions

B. Adjunctive Psychotherapy
   1. important of continuing and monitoring lithium treatment
   2. build better family and social relationships
   3. teaching bipolar patients about their disorder
   4. help clients develop solutions for difficulties brought on by disorder

III. Treatments for Mood Disorders: The State of the Field

A. Most Treatable of Mental Disorders

B. Unipolar Patterns Reduced or Eliminated in 2 to 20 Weeks

C. Lithium (Often Combined with Counseling) is Treatment of Choice for Bipolar

D. May Be Various Kinds of Unipolar Depression

E. Different Depression Patterns Might Be Matched to Kinds of Treatments

Learning Objectives:
1. Describe the prognosis for person with mood disorders in treatment.
2. Explain the psychodynamic approach to treating clients with unipolar depression.
3. Describe behavioral techniques for depressed clients.
4. Describe and evaluate interpersonal therapy (IPT) for depressed clients.
5. List the four phases of cognitive treatment for depression and evaluate its effectiveness.
6. Describe electroconvulsive therapy and explain its effects on neurotransmitters.
7. Compare and contrast MAO inhibitors and tricyclics.
8. Distinguish between traditional tricyclics and new second-generation antidepressants.
9. Summarize the effectiveness of the various treatments for unipolar depression.
10. Describe the role of lithium in treating bipolar depression.

Instruction Suggestions:
1. *Mini-Lecture.* **Applying Karen Horney's Ideas to Depression**
   Karen Horney viewed the core of insecurities as basic anxiety, which developed due to inadequacies in the parent-child relationship. These inadequacies could be experiencing too little nurturance, too much rejection and hostility, being overwhelmed and smothered without a chance to develop oneself, and a number of other imbalances in the relationship.

   As a result, people learn to protect their vulnerable and anxious selves by adapting one of three exaggerated interpersonal relationships. Some people *move toward* people and become overdependent on them. These people are especially prone to depression because a real or imagined loss disturbs their basic way of coping with insecurities. They cannot imagine how they will be able to cope without relying on the person who is lost or anticipated to become lost to them. They are depressed about their own unworthiness and basic inadequacy and then doubly depressed because they lose a person who helps them cope in spite of their personal shortcomings.

   Others *move away* from people. They protect the vulnerable self by not allowing themselves to get close to others. As a result, they limit their own experience of many socially reinforcing situations. Having below average reinforcers is one cause of depression.

   Still others *move against* people. Like the group above, they may become depressed due to fewer reinforcers in their lives. Moreover, their general pattern is to be hostile toward others. If they apply this same hostile alienation toward themselves, then they experience greater depression, as one way to define depression is "anger turned inward."

   In different words, perhaps, both the cognitive therapy and IPT address some of Horney's ideas during treatment. Can you find some of these parallels?

2. *Class Discussion.* A good topic to discuss is that of Freud and Abraham's parallel between depression and grief. Have students describe personal situations that fit this model. Point out that all depression and grief involves a sense of loss. Then have them compare the similarities and differences between the losses of a divorced person and a widowed person. How are their emotional and behavioral reactions the same or different? Do students admit that they have "grieved" over grades or college admissions? Do people

grieve job losses as well as people losses? If your students were to erect tombstones for lost dreams, situations, opportunities, and anything "non-people deaths," what would they bury in the cemetery? What rituals could help in dealing with these "deaths"?

3. *Class Discussion.* Ask the class to compare personal effectiveness training and psychodrama.

4. *Class Activity.* As a class or in small groups, "brainstorm" a list of things that students experiencing mild depression could do (in the context of this college) to help reduce the depression (e.g., take a walk, do some good deed for another person, meditate, make a tape of good, "up" music, start feeding birds each day).

5. *Lecture Additions.* Introduce students to O.H. Mowrer's *"You Are Your Secrets"* from *The New Group Therapy.* The basic idea is that when people are alone, they often think about their secrets. Since most people keep "bad things" secret, when they think about these things they get depressed. Therefore, Mowrer suggests that we should learn to be open and honest about our negative characteristics and behaviors so they cannot haunt us when alone. In addition, one should anonymously do small, affordable good deeds for others. These good deeds then become one's secrets, and when alone one can feel good about them. Mowrer got this idea from the novel *The Magnificent Obsession.*

6. *Class Demonstration.* Try to show one or more ECT scene from a movie (e.g., *One Flew Over the Cuckoo's Nest*) and also from a documentary. Discuss the similarities and differences in the ECT shown in the movie and in the documentary. Discuss reactions to the treatment.

7. *Class Demonstration.* Ask a pharmacist or psychiatrist to speak about psychoactive drugs for depression, and how some medicines can contribute to depression.

8. *Class Discussion.* Share some of the controversy over Prozac's side effects. Discuss how all drugs have side effects, and how some medicines can contribute to depression.

9. *Class Demonstration.* Have a counselor come to class to address issues of how therapists deal with the stresses of hearing and dealing with the problems of other people. Are they affected by depression of others? How do they work through these feelings? What do they think are the most effective counseling techniques when dealing with depression? Do they incorporate a number of these strategies into their own lives? You might have students write questions on file cards and give these to your speaker to address. You might want to use a campus counselor who can specifically address concerns of depression among students.

10. *Class Demonstration.* Take the time to research your state's laws about ECT and to get an ECT consent form from a local hospital. You might call local hospitals and find out how frequently they utilize ECT. Use this specific information in conjunction with Box 9-3, which addresses more general issues about ECT and the law. Using Table 9-3, have students discuss whether they might agree to ECT if they were severely depressed.

11. *Class Demonstration.* Bring a *Physician's Desk Reference (PDR)* to class and look up information, especially side effects, for the drugs that reduce depression given in Table 9-4. Ask students for their reactions to this material.

Topic Overview:

I. Suicide Statistics

  A. Only Humans Knowingly End Their Own Lives

  B. Prevalence
    1. one of top ten causes of death in Western society
    2. 120,000 deaths annually; 30,000 in the United States
    3. more than 2 million parasuicides (attempts not resulting in death) annually; 600,000 in the United States
    4. over 5,000,000 living Americans have survived a suicide attempt
    5. because suicide is stigmatizing, the statistics are probably low and some suicides are classified as accidents
    6. suicide is not a DSM-III-R mental disorder but at least half of all suicides are associated with mental disorders, especially mood disorders, substance abuse, and schizophrenia

  C. Misconceptions About Suicide Are Common

II. What Is Suicide?

  A. Defining Suicide
    1. intentional, direct, and conscious effort to end one's life
    2. death seekers have a clear intentions of ending their lives at the time of their attempt, therefore are more likely to use lethal means
    3. death initiators want to end their lives because they believe they are already dying and just hastening the process
    4. death ignorers do not believe they are ending their existence but going to a better existence, and is typical of child suicides and religious adults
    5. death darers are ambivalent in their intention to die and are most likely to take actions that do not guarantee death
    6. subintentional deaths are deaths in which individuals were indirect, covert, partial, or unconscious in their acts, such as in mismanaging medicines
    7. in addition to Shneidman's categories above, Karl Menninger added a category of chronic suicide, or people who behave in life-endangering ways over an extended period of time

  B. The Study of Suicide
    1. hard to study because subjects are now dead
    2. use retrospective analysis, or a psychological autopsy
    3. less than a quarter of all suicide victims have been in counseling and fewer than 15% leave suicide notes

C. Patterns and Statistics
1. suicide rates vary in different nations—highest: Hungary, Austria, West Germany, Denmark, Finland, Switzerland, Sweden (all over 20 per 100,000)
2. low rates: Egypt, Mexico, Italy, Ireland, Israel, Greece, Spain (less than 9 per 100,000)
3. United States and Canada at about 13 per 100,000
4. religious affiliations and beliefs partially account for national differences with Catholic, Jewish, and Muslim countries lower (exception: Roman Catholic Austria has high rate)
5. women make three times as many attempts but men die from suicide three times as often
6. men use more violent methods (e.g., shooting, stabbing, hanging) than women (e.g., barbiturates) and may also be clearer in their intent to die
7. married persons have lower rate, divorced persons have the highest rate
8. whites have much higher rate than blacks or Hispanics but Native Americans have a very high rate

III. Precipitating Factors in Suicide

A. Stressful Events and Situations
1. more undesirable events recently among suicide attempters than others
2. suicide attempts may be precipitated by a single recent event or a series
3. common precipitating event is loss of a loved one by death, divorce, breakup, rejection
4. common factor is painful or disabling illness
5. victims of abusive or repressive environments who have little or no hope of escape are at risk
6. jobs with higher risks include psychiatrists, psychologists, physicians, dentists, lawyers, unskilled laborers
7. linked to suicide is role conflict

B. Mood and Thought Changes
1. many attempts preceded by a shift in mood
2. most commonly an increase in sadness
3. but also anxiety, anger, or shame
4. single most sensitive indicator of suicidal intent is a sense of hopelessness
5. a pattern of dichotomous thinking; problems and solutions are viewed as either-or

C. Alcohol Use
1. studies show 20-90% of those who commit suicide consume alcohol just before their act
2. alcohol's disinhibiting effect may allow contemplating suicide, overcome fears, and lower prohibitions against violence

D. Mental Disorders
1. not all who attempt suicide are mentally ill
2. 30-70% display a mental disorder

3. most common: mood disorders, substance use disorders (especially alcoholism), and schizophrenia (about 10-15% of each disorder make suicide attempts)
4. because more have mood disorders, more suicide attempts from this disorder than the others
5. suicidal thoughts part of major depressive disorder syndrome
6. among those severely depressed, suicide risk increases as mood improves because of getting enough energy to make an attempt

E. Modeling: The Contagion of Suicide
1. more people try to commit suicide after observing or reading about a suicide
2. suicides by entertainers and political figures are followed by increase in numbers of suicides
3. highly publicized accounts may trigger suicides, although most victims have histories of emotional problems
4. suicides in a school, workplace, or small community may trigger other attempts

IV. Views on Suicide

A. The Psychodynamic View
1. usually result from depression and self-directed anger and hatred
2. Stekel (1910) said, "No one kills himself who has not wanted to kill another or at least wished the death of another"
3. Freud's basic death instinct, Thanatos
4. relationship between childhood losses and later suicidal behaviors
5. national suicide rates drop significantly in times of war, which means a redirection of self-destructive energy to destruction against others

B. The Biological View
1. pedigree studies show higher rates of suicidal behavior among the parents and close relatives of suicidal persons
2. people who commit suicide often have low levels of serotonin
3. the link between low serotonin and suicide is not necessarily mediated by depression; low levels among suicidal subjects with no history of depression and among attempters with personality disorders, schizophrenia, anxiety disorders, and substance dependence
4. low serotonin levels and strong aggressive impulses may be the suicidal combination

C. The Sociocultural View
1. in 1897, Durkheim developed the first comprehensive theory of suicidal behavior
2. egoistic suicides committed by people over whom society has little or no control, i.e., by loners who are isolated, alienated, and nonreligious
3. altruistic suicides are well-integrated persons who sacrifice their lives for the well-being of society
4. anomic suicides are committed by persons whose social environment is unstable and who feel let down by society
5. societies go through periods of anomie and have correspondingly high suicide rates

6. change in immediate surroundings rather than general society can lead to anomic suicide
7. Durkheim's theory does not explain why some but not a majority of those experiencing anomie commit suicide

V. Suicide in Different Age Groups

A. Children
1. relatively infrequent but increasing
2. about 300 children under 15 years annually in the United States
3. boys three times as likely as girls to kill themselves
4. most typical is overdose of drugs at home while living with one parent and with at least one previous attempt
5. often preceded by behavior patterns such as running away, accidents, temper tantrums, self-deprecation, loneliness, psychophysiological illness
6. because of cognitive limitations usually death ignorers
7. suicidal thinking is more common than once thought

B. Adolescents and Young Adults
1. suicidal actions much more common after 14 than before
2. in United States, more than 6,000 adolescents and young adults kill themselves yearly
3. suicide is third leading cause of death (after accidents, homicides)
4. highest among whites but rate of increase faster now for black youths
5. one-third of teenagers have considered suicide
6. warning signs: tiredness, sleep loss, loss of appetite, mood changes, decline in school performance, increased substance use, withdrawal, increased letter writing, giving away possessions
7. most common is drug overdose but more deaths from shootings
8. most often at home after school
9. about half linked to clinical depression
10. stress at school—either keeping up or perfectionistic achievement
11. struggling with anger
12. make more incomplete attempts than older persons
13. among 18-24 years, higher for college students than others
14. among college students, experiences of academic pressures, loss of social support, unresolved older problems interacting with college situations, unknown resources
15. suicide rate for adolescents and young adults is high and increasing due to increased competition for jobs, colleges, and athletic honors, world politics and nuclear war possibilities, and availability and use of drugs

C. The Elderly
1. the most likely to commit suicide (22 of 100,000)
2. factors: illness, loss of close friends and relatives, loss of control over one's life, loss of societal status, increased hopelessness, loneliness, depression
3. risk high in first year of bereavement for a spouse
4. more resolute and more suicide attempts are completed
5. lower among minority groups and especially elderly Native Americans

VI. Treatment and Suicide

    A. Treatment after a Suicide Attempt
        1. first, medical care
        2. many do not become involved in therapy
        3. outpatient therapy
        4. behavior therapy has faster improvement but insight therapy also helps

    B. Suicide Prevention
        1. first suicide prevention program was Farberow and Shneidman's Los Angeles Suicide Prevention Center in 1955
        2. see suicidal people as people in crisis
        3. most counselors are paraprofessionals
        4. goals: establishing a positive relationship, understanding and clarifying the problem, assessing suicide potential, assessing and mobilizing the caller's resources, formulating a plan

    C. The Effectiveness of Suicide Prevention
        1. mixed study results
        2. only 2% of people who actually killed themselves in Lost Angeles ever contacted the prevention center
        3. does seem to avert suicide for high-risk people who do call
        4. least informed of professionals who might be contacted by suicidal persons seems to be the clergy

VII. Suicide

    A. Suicide as Publicized Topic

    B. Know Much About Motivations, Conditions, and Risk Factors

    C. Public Education about Suicide

    D. Need Better, More Comprehensive Explanations of Causes

    E. Need Better, More Successful Interventions

Learning Objectives:
1. Define suicide and know how common suicide is.
2. Describe each of the four kinds of people who intentionally end their lives: death seeker, death initiator, death ignorer, and death darer. Also describe the category of subintentional death.
3. Describe the research strategies of retrospective analysis and interviewing suicide survivors.
4. Know the effects of cultural aspects, race, and sex on suicide rates.
5. Be familiar with common precipitating factors of suicide.
6. List four long-term stresses that increase the frequency of suicide.
7. Discuss how mood changes, hopelessness, and dichotomous thinking are related to suicide.
8. Know which mental disorders are linked most strongly to suicide.

9. Describe the kinds of models that trigger suicides.
10. Give the psychodynamic explanation for suicide, including the role of Thanatos.
11. Give the biological role of suicide, including explaining the role of serotonin.
12. Compare and contrast Durkheim's three categories of suicide: egoistic, altruistic, anomic.
13. Discuss age differences in suicidal thought and action.
14. Discuss the reasons for the increasing rates of suicides in adolescents and young adults in recent years.
15. Explain the high suicide rate among the elderly.
16. Describe therapy for suicide survivors.
17. Discuss characteristics of suicide prevention programs.

Instruction Suggestions:
1. *Class Activity.* Write on the blackboard "Suicide is _____." Ask students to write down five ways to complete this sentence and collect their answers. Read some of them out loud. Students may write things such as "...a permanent solution to a temporary crisis," "...saying no thanks, world," "a waste of humanity," "a way to get on with karma," "a mess left for one's heirs," and so forth. Discuss what the responses say about values and societal beliefs.

2. *Class Demonstration.* The chapter provides the statistic "At least 60 Americans will kill themselves by this time tomorrow." An effective way to start a lecture on suicide is to translate statistics to how many will kill themselves during the time of this one lecture. For example, if your class time is one hour, write 3-1/2 and 68-1/2 on the board. Then say, "By the time this class period is over, 3-1/2 Americans will have killed themselves and at least 68-1/2 will have made attempts on their lives."

3. *Class Discussion.* When discussing Shneidman's kinds of suicides, discuss what might be the primary values held by people whose suicide attempts fit each of these categories. This can also be done while discussing Durkheim's classification of suicides.

4. *Class Discussion.* Discuss the accuracy of statistics about suicide. For example, might some national statistics be adjusted to better fit cultural beliefs and values? Or how often are accidents listed instead of suicides to spare mourners? Or, are there times when suicides are actually overestimated (e.g., might family members want accidental death from hanging for masturbatory purposes listed as suicide, or might anti-abortion supporters want to overestimate the number of deaths due to distress over having an abortion?)?

5. *Class Activity.* Should newspaper obituaries list suicide as cause of death? Generate a list of advantages (e.g., only way to work on ending the stigma that is still is attached, might indicate to others that there is need for more mental health services) and disadvantages (e.g., added grief to family members, might encourage other suicides).

6. *Mini-Lecture.* **Speculations on Gender Roles and Suicide Attempts**
Do gender roles influence suicidal attempts? The book suggests that men are more familiar with guns and more willing to use this violent method against themselves than are women. Do gender roles influence other aspects of suicide? It has been proposed that men get more negative responses from a failed suicide attempt (e.g., "Gee, he isn't even man enough to kill himself"), while women are more likely to get sympathy and help. This might be one reason why women make so many more attempts than men.

Women are more likely to be in charge of cleaning, and police officers have noted that women who kill themselves are more likely to have considered what survivors will have to deal with because of the suicide. One officer related an incident in which a woman who shot herself apparently first cleaned the entire house, did her family's laundry and laid out directions for how the kids should dress themselves the next week, and spread newspapers out on the kitchen floor so that it would be easier to clean up her blood.

Other professionals who have found bodies have also commented that women place more attention on how the body will look. They often choose their clothing carefully, or even choose to die nude. They may be more likely to use pills because they will die without disfigurement and will look like they died peacefully—often with carefully done makeup.

What other speculations can you think of about how men and women take their gender roles to the grave?

7. *Class Demonstration.* Many appropriate speakers are possible to invite to talk about what they have seen and experienced in their careers in relationship to suicide. You could even compose a panel. Consider the following persons: a medical examiner/coroner, a suicide crisis line worker, emergency room personnel, a counselor, a police officer, a member of the clergy, a funeral director, a suicide survivor. Have them describe their experiences or work, their values about suicide, how they deal with survivors and family members, and how they come to terms with the emotional aspects of their work.

8. *Class Discussion.* Have students describe examples of mass suicide and their reactions to them. You might want to compare and contrast the mass suicide of Jim Jones' cult followers in Jonestown and the suicide of the Jewish school girls who chose group suicide when they learned that Hitler was going to force them to be prostitutes.

9. *Class Discussion.* Discuss reasons for the popularity of the book *The Final Exit*, which describes the best ways to kill oneself. Discuss the virtues or non-virtues of the Hemlock Society, which promotes safe, self-chosen suicide. You might want to bring in the book or the society's newsletter and possibly share an excerpt. What do these materials and this group say about our societal values? You might also want to bring in a discussion of legal active euthanasia, such as in Holland, where patient and family doctor can agree to a medically caused death.

10. *Class Discussion.* Ask the class to discuss their beliefs about suicide cults among teenagers. If they believe that they exist, ask them to describe their purpose, how they get going, how they might lower inhibitions about committing suicide while also providing information about how to kill oneself. What could be done to counteract cults?

11. *Class Discussion.* Discuss the role of rock lyrics in suicides among teenagers. Do they think that a rock group could be held responsible for a death that occurs after a young person has repeatedly listened to their morbid, suicide-praising lyrics? What role might games like Dungeons and Dragons play in suicides among children and adolescents? Movie plots? Would you censor these aspects of culture?

12. *Class Activity.* Create a one-day workshop for college students that is designed to inform them about suicide and related factors. What topics would you cover? What resources would you point out? What kinds of handouts would you like to have?

13. *Lecture Additions.* Discuss specific cases of altruistic suicides, such as the deaths of three young people after the Soviet Coup in 1991. What motivated these three? How was history affected? What was the society's response? Other examples include Kent State campus during the Vietnam War and Vietnamese Buddhist monks who immolated themselves to protest the war. For what causes would students be willing to die?

14. *Class Activity.* Design a grief counseling treatment program targeted for survivors of suicide. What aspects would you include, and why?

Topic Overview:
I. Factitious Disorders with Physical Symptoms

    A. Definitions
        1. malingering is intentionally feigning illness to achieve external gains
        2. factitious disorder with physical symptoms is intentionally producing physical symptoms so that the sick role can meet internal psychological needs

    B. Characteristics
        1. total fabrication, self-inflicted, or exaggeration of physical condition
        2. dramatic medical history but vague when pressed for details
        3. extensive knowledge of medical terminology
        4. demand attention from hospital staff and may be eager to undergo painful testing or treatment, even surgery
        5. if confronted with the pattern, patients offer denials and then rapidly discharge themselves and go to another medical facility
        6. in Munchausen syndrome, persons go from hospital to hospital reciting symptoms, getting admitted, and receiving treatment
        7. prevalence is not known
        8. more common among men than among women
        9. another version is factitious disorder with psychological symptoms, in which people feign symptoms suggestive of mental disorders, especially psychosis

  II. Somatoform Disorders

    A. Hysterical Somatoform Disorders
        1. involve altered or lost physical functioning without organic base
        2. conversion disorder is a loss of physical functioning in one or more areas due to psychological conflict or need
        3. most dramatic are neurological dysfunctioning, e.g., paralysis, seizures, blindness, anesthesia, aphonia
        4. can also be autonomic, endocrine, or cardiopulmonary dysfunctioning
        5. mostly late adolescence or young adulthood and more women than men
        6. somatization disorder, or Briquet's syndrome, is having 13 or more physical ailments without organic basis over a long period of time
        7. about 1% of women and rarely any men receive this diagnosis
        8. pain with no medical explanation can be somatoform pain disorder, diagnosed more with women than men and more in middle age and up
        9. somatoform pain disorder often begins after an accident or during an illness
      10. often *la belle indifférence* with hysterical disorders
      11. symptoms of hysterical disorders might not correspond to neurological anatomy

12. hysteria often involves selectivity of symptoms or inconsistency

B. Preoccupation Somatoform Disorders
   1. take minimal physical symptoms as signs of serious physical problems
   2. those with hypochondriasis unrealistically and fearfully interpret minor physical discomforts as signs of serious illness
   3. high anxiety and minor bodily symptoms is hypochondriasis and more bodily symptoms and lower anxiety is somatization disorder
   4. hypochondriasis mostly emerges between 20 and 30
   5. hypochondriasis equal among men and women
   6. two types of hypochondriacal patients are hostile and dependent
   7. body dysmorphic disorder or dysmorphophobia involves preoccupation with imagined or exaggerated defect in appearance

C. Views on Somatoform Disorders
   1. current beliefs about hysterical ailments go back to late nineteenth century
   2. Freud's psychoanalytic theory began with his account of hysterical symptoms
   3. because of response to hypnosis, Freud thought hysteria was a conversion of emotional conflicts into physical symptoms
   4. somatoform disorders have both primary gain and secondary gain
   5. cognitive view is that conversion communicates some distressing emotion into a "language" familiar to the patient
   6. sick role may distract person from own psychological pain while allowing message to others about their great distress
   7. behaviorists believe the physical symptoms of hysterical disorders bring rewards
   8. the role of an invalid has much secondary gain

D. Treatments for Somatoform Disorders
   1. seek counseling as a last resort
   2. exposure and response-prevention interventions for preoccupation somatoform disorders
   3. insight, suggestion, or confrontation for hysterical somatoform disorders
   4. conversion disorders and somatoform pain disorders respond better to counseling than somatization disorders
   5. problem is that a physical illness might have been missed, especially difficult ones such as multiple sclerosis, systematic lupus erythematosis

III. Psychophysiological Disorders

A. "Traditional" Psychophysiological Disorders
   1. during first half of century, psychophysiological disorders organized by affected body system
   2. ulcers are lesions or holes in stomach or duodenum wall resulting in pain, burning, and sometimes vomiting and bleeding and caused by interaction of psychological factors, environmental stress and anger, and dependent personality
   3. asthma, a leading cause of illness among the young, is the constriction of body's airways and caused by generalized anxiety, heightened dependency needs, environmental stress, and troubled family relationships
   4. chronic muscle contraction headaches or tension headaches

5. migraine headaches are caused by pattern of constriction of blood vessels and are most likely to occur right after stress
6. essential hypertension, or high blood pressure, is associated with constant environmental danger, chronic anger, and unexpressed need for power
7. coronary heart disease involves angina pectoris, coronary occlusion, and myocardial infarction
8. Schwartz's disregulation model deals with problems in the negative feedback loops, such as environmental overload, faulty environment information processing, malfunctioning peripheral organ, or failed feedback mechanisms
9. environmental factors leading to disregulation: cataclysmic, personal, background stressors
10. certain needs, attitudes, emotions may increase odds for psychophysiological disorders, such as dependency or unresolved anger
11. type A personality is driven, hostile, cynical, impatient, competitive, ambitious
12. type A associated with coronary heart disease
13. role of the sympathetic and parasympathetic divisions of the autonomic nervous system (ANS)
14. Seyle's general adaptation syndrome: alarm stage, resistance stage, exhaustion stage
15. role of pituitary-adrenal endocrine system
16. local somatic weaknesses, or specific organics that are defective or prone to dysfunction under stress
17. role of individual response specificity, such as repeated activation of a "favored" system, may wear it down
18. organ dysfunctioning from autonomic learning, or conditioning of autonomic nervous system
19. added psychophysical disorders: irritable bowel syndrome, psoriasis, eczema, rheumatoid arthritis, hypoglycemia

B. "New" Psychophysiological Disorders
  1. stress may make one vulnerable to viral and bacterial infections
  2. Holmes and Rahe's 1967 Social Adjustment Rating Scale showed that the more recent life changes, the more health problems
  3. sudden death with a psychological trauma is not uncommon
  4. bereavement stress can be fatal
  5. new field of psychoneuroimmunology
  6. immune system provides protection from antigens by lymphocytes
  7. types of lymphocytes: helper T-cells, killer T-cells, and B-cells
  8. stress can interfere with the activity of lymphocytes
  9. during stress, people may stay healthy on the surface but changes in the immune system increase susceptibility to illness
  10. increased autonomic arousal can also suppress immune system
  11. perceptions of stress rather than actual level determines vulnerability
  12. "hardy" personality style takes on challenge and takes control in living
  13. inhibited power motive style related to immunologic dysfunctioning

C. Psychological Treatments for Psychological Disorders
  1. need field of behavioral medicine
  2. relaxation training to prevent or treat illnesses related to stress and heightened autonomic functioning

3. biofeedback training moderately helpful with anxiety disorders and physical disorders
4. meditation may be helpful and has been shown to help treat hypertension, cardiovascular problems, and viral infections
5. hypnosis helpful in treating pain, and researchers have shown its role in preventing bacterial and viral infections
6. stress inoculation may help coping with chronic and severe pain disorders
7. insight psychotherapy may help general levels of anxiety
8. psychological interventions most helpful combined with other techniques and medical treatments

IV. Psychological Factors and Physical Disorders: The State of the Field

    A. Psychology Becoming More Involved

    B. Increase in Research Studies

    C. Increase in Relaxation Training and Cognitive Therapy

    D. Understanding of Interrelationship of Brain and Body

Learning Objectives:
1. Evaluate the current view of mind-body interaction, or dualism.
2. Define factitious disorders and describe Munchausen syndrome.
3. Distinguish between somatoform disorders and factitious disorders.
4. Describe each of the hysterical somatoform disorders: conversion disorders, somatization disorders, and somatoform pain disorders.
5. Explain how diagnosticians distinguish hysterical somatoform disorders from the medical disorders.
6. Describe the preoccupation somatoform disorders of hypochondriasis and body dysmorphic disorders and explain typical treatment.
7. Compare the features of psychodynamic, cognitive, and behavioral treatments for hysterical disorders.
8. Define psychophysiological disorders and describe typical kinds.
9. Describe the disregulation model of psychophysiological disorders and identify three general contributing factors.
10. Explain Hans Seyle's general adaptation syndrome.
11. Define the concepts of local somatic weaknesses, individual response specificity, and autonomic learning.
12. Describe the psychoneuroimmunology area of study.
13. List and explain various interventions used in behavioral medicine.

Instruction Suggestions:
1. *Class Discussion.* Should children with serious illness (perhaps terminal illness) be told directly and honestly about their health condition? Are there situations in which you would not tell children that they were seriously sick? A study of 117 childhood cancer survivors and their families found that families thought children should be told early using honest language that the child can comprehend, and told how to have mastery over the disease.

2. *Lecture Additions.* Type A behaviors are displayed by some children as well as by many adult Americans. Researchers suggest that children as young as three years can exhibit a marked pattern of impatience and restlessness (e.g., much squirming and sighing), expectation of high standards for themselves, and above average competition. Children may carry these behaviors with them into adulthood with their eventual impact on health factors. Currently, little is known about the role of genetic factors and temperament on early Type A behaviors, but research suggests that parent-child interactions influence Type A level of children. In one study, mothers of Type A boys provided fewer positive evaluations of their sons' performances than did other mothers. Therefore, these sons may make themselves work harder, more competitively, and more anxiously in order to receive their mothers' approval.

3. *Mini-lecture.* **Close-Up Look At Asthma**
Asthma, a common respiratory illness involving the airway obstruction from degranulation of mast cells in the lung's lining, is underdiagnosed and therefore undertreated. It is sometimes misdiagnosed as recurrent bronchitis or pneumonia. About 10% of all children have asthma—about 3.2 American children. Asthma is also prevalent among adults (there are nearly 10 million asthmatic Americans), but 80% of those with asthma experienced their first symptoms before they were five years old.

Asthma can be affected by many conditions—an inherited genetic predisposition, viral infections, food allergens, inhaled allergens, exercise, climatic changes, cigarette smoke, pets, and emotional stress. Research has shown that passive smoking also increases problems with asthma.

Three commonly held misconceptions about asthma are that:
    (1) Asthma means being fragile and not being able to participate in gym class. In fact, 11% of the athletes on U.S. Olympic teams have asthma.
    (2) Asthma is outgrown. Actually, only half experience a remission of symptoms during puberty.
    (3) Emotions cause asthma. Stress affects asthma but is not the primary cause.

4. *Class Activity.* Have the class create a list of the advantages of being sick. What childhood messages did students get about being sick? As students (e.g., allowed excuse for missing test)? What messages were received about good health? About one's own role in controlling one's health?

5. *Class Project.* If there is a pain clinic nearby, arrange to take your class for a visit.

6. *Class Demonstration.* Have a professional who works with pain speak to the class. Possibilities include an accupuncturist, a chiropractor, an osteopathic doctor who does manipulation, a neurologist, a behavioral counselor who does pain management.

7. *Class Discussion.* Many mental disorders involve illness and physical symptoms—

somatoform disorders, psychophysiological disorders, and so forth. Why aren't there any categories for those who are overly concerned with good health—the "health nuts of the world"—aren't they the flipside of hypochondriasis?

8. *Lecture Additions.* Some psychologists, when reading all the research on Type A and health, are much less concerned than previously about the effects of Type A. Although Type As have a higher rate of CHD, their personality style also helps them to survive their heart attacks more than others who have heart attacks.

9. *Class Activity.* Have class members take the Holmes & Rahe Scale and turn in the "number" of LCUs. Provide statistical information about the class's LCUs—the range, mean, median, and mode. Does it form a normal curve? You may wish to collect more specific data anonymously and relate the most common and least common stressors for students in the class. You can suggest what life changes could be added as students and try to assign an appropriate number of LCUs per addition. You can also incorporate Box 11-2 into this activity and make a list of common student hassles and uplifts.

10. *Class Discussion.* Have the class discuss the relationship between health and academic stress. Do health problems fit a semester pattern?

11. *Class Demonstration.* Have an AIDS patient, AIDS health worker, or other relevant speaker come to class and address the psychological effects of HIV and AIDS.

12. *Class Discussion.* Discuss students' beliefs about their own role in health and sickness. Can they affect the course of their disease? Can they do things that prevent diseases? Is it the patient's fault for being ill?

Topic Overview:
I. Anorexia Nervosa

A. Characteristic Symptoms According to DSM-III-R
1. intense fear of gaining weight or becoming fat
2. refusal to maintain body weight above minimal normal weight
3. body image distortion and disturbance
4. amenorrhea for at least three consecutive cycles

B. Incidence
1. 95% females
2. peak age of 14 and 18 years, but can be any age
3. typically begins after a slightly overweight female decides to lose a few pounds
4. often follows a stressful event, parental separation, moving away, personal failure
5. 5-18% die from this disorder
6. incidence on the increase

C. The Pursuit of Thinness and Fear of Obesity
1. being thin is life's central goal
2. also called a "weight phobia"
3. half reduce weight by restricting food intake
4. thinness as a personal test of self-discipline
5. lose weight by vomiting or abusing laxatives and diuretics (bulimia nervosa)
6. in constant motion, which hides fatigue
7. following a rigid regimen of exercise
8. little interest in sexual activities

D. Cognitive Disturbances
1. low opinion of their body shape and physical attractiveness due to distorted body image and overestimating body size
2. anorexics tend to overestimate their body size, while others tend to underestimate their body size
3. difficult to identify internal sensations of hunger and satiety and report being full after eating only a small amount
4. fail to recognize fatigue, body temperature changes, and emotions, often confusing emotions with other sensations
5. development of maladaptive attitudes and misperceptions centering on perfection, self-control, self-discipline, and weight and body shape

E. Preoccupation with Food
   1. much thinking about, planning for, and reading about food
   2. may be result of food deprivation or a contributing cause

F. Personality and Mood Problems
   1. at least mildly depressed and low self-esteem
   2. anxiety, general indecisiveness, poor concentration, and specific fears about body weight
   3. sleep disorders, e.g., insomnia
   4. obsessive compulsive patterns of behavior

G. Medical Problems
   1. amenorrhea
   2. lowered body temperature, low blood pressure, body swelling, slow heart rate
   3. metabolic and electrolyte imbalances that can lead to cardiac arrest, congestive heart failure, or circulatory collapse
   4. severe nutritional deficiencies can result in changes in skin appearance, brittle nails, cold and blue hands and feet, lost hair, lanugo
   5. drive for thinness and fear of obesity leads to self-starvation, which leads to preoccupation with food and resulting increases in anxiety, depression, obsessive rigidity, and medical dysfunctioning

II. Bulimia Nervosa

A. Central Characteristics
   1. "bulimia" comes from Greek for "cattle hunger," symbolizing that food is hardly tasted during binges
   2. other names: binge-purge syndrome, gorge-purge syndrome, dietary chaos syndrome
   3. recurrent episodes of binge eating
   4. feeling of lack of control over eating behavior during eating binges
   5. habitual recourse to self-induced vomiting, use of laxatives or diuretics, strict dieting or fasting, vigorous exercise
   6. persistent overconcern with body shape and weight
   7. bulimic anorexia nervosa is a combination of bulimia nervosa and anorexia nervosa

B. Clinical Picture
   1. secretive, rapid eating of massive amounts of food
   2. sweet foods with high caloric content and soft texture
   3. early on, binges triggered by upsetting events, hunger, boredom
   4. later, binges become carefully planned events
   5. binges begin with feelings of unbearable tension
   6. during binge, person feels unable to stop eating
   7. binge followed by extreme self-reproach, guilt, depression, fear of weight gain
   8. binges average 2,000 to 4,000 calories and bulimics average 12 binge episodes weekly (or 14 hours)
   9. "purging" is trying to undo the effects of the binge and repeated vomiting disrupts the body's satiety mechanisms
   10. purging is reinforced by immediate sense of relief and being able to remove "threatening" foods and maintain an acceptable appearance

C. Bulimia Nervosa (BN) versus Anorexia Nervosa (AN)
   1. both develop after a period of intense dieting
   2. both fear becoming obese and are driven to be thin
   3. both preoccupied with food, weight, and appearance
   4. both experience depression and anxiety and feel the need to be perfect
   5. both believe they do weigh too much
   6. both have difficulty identifying and differentiating internal states
   7. BN more likely to recognize they display a pathological pattern
   8. BN more inclined to trust others and to want to please others
   9. AN less interested in sex and less sexually experienced
   10. AN more obsessive
   11. BN more dramatic mood swings
   12. BN less able to control impulses
   13. BN medical complications include dental problems, hypokalemia leading to
       weakness, gastrointestinal disorders, paralysis, kidney disease, irregular heart
       rhythms, heart damage, also damaged esophagus wall

III. Explanations of Eating Disorders

A. Sociocultural Pressures
   1. Western society's current emphasis on thinness and standards of attractiveness
   2. more in upper socioeconomic classes
   3. prejudice and hostility against overweight people
   4. although extreme obesity is unhealthy, mild or moderate obesity is not

B. Family Environment
   1. families that emphasize thinness, physical appearance, and dieting
   2. abnormal and confusing family interactions and forms of communication
   3. enmeshed family patterns, or overinvolved with each others' lives and welfare and
      not speaking about one's own ideas and feelings
   4. enmeshed families are affectionate and loyal but they foster dependency and
      clinging, with parents too involved in their children's lives
   5. enmeshed families had difficulty dealing with adolescent needs to be independent,
      so teen often takes on a sick role
   6. mixed research results on enmeshed families
   7. higher-than-average levels of stress and conflict and poorer problem-solving skills
      with members supporting each other less and criticizing, rejecting, and competing

C. Ego Deficiencies and Cognitive Disturbances
   1. Bruch said that disturbed mother-child interactions lead to serious ego deficiencies
      in the child, such as poor sense of autonomy and control, and to severe perceptual
      and other cognitive disturbances
   2. effective parents provide discriminating attention to their children's biological and
      emotional needs but ineffective parents impose their own definitions of needs on the
      children
   3. unable to rely on internal standards, children use external guides and are viewed as
      "model children"
   4. learn to do things that please family but fail to develop genuine self-reliance

5. as adolescents, don't know how to establish needed autonomy so overcome sense of helplessness by achieving extreme self-control
6. people with eating disorders perceive and distinguish internal cues inaccurately and end up "feeding" their emotions

D. Biological Factors
   1. bulimia nervosa associated with a heightened physiological need for carbohydrates
   2. lateral hypothalamus produces hunger and ventromedial hypothalamus depresses hunger
   3. weight set point influences body's metabolic rate
   4. weight set point is range of body weight (percent of body fat) that is normal as determined by genetic inheritance, early eating practices, and need for internal equilibrium
   5. strict diets modify the set point and sets hyperlipogenesis into motion

E. Mood Disorders
   1. higher rates of depression, sadness, low self-esteem, pessimism, logic errors
   2. high rate of those with an eating disorder have a clinical major depression
   3. close relatives of those with eating disorders have high rate of mood disorders
   4. often have low activity of serotonin
   5. some anti-depressants useful in altering dysfunctional eating patterns

F. Multidimensional Perspective
   1. predispositions, precipitants, and perpetuators
   2. an interaction causes eating disorders
   3. need to know what the protective factors are as well as vulnerable factors

IV. Treatments for Eating Disorders

A. Treatments for Anorexia Nervosa
   1. increase caloric intake and get quick weight gain
   2. in life-threatening cases, use tube and intravenous feedings
   3. antipsychotic drugs can be used to reverse starvation habits and antidepressant medications useful in relieving depression and obsessions
   4. operant conditioning approaches
   5. supportive nursing care combined with a high-calorie diet
   6. addressing underlying problems and altering maladaptive thinking patterns
   7. awareness of autonomy issues
   8. activity programs such as artwork
   9. help clients to recognize and trust their own feelings, especially by self-discovery
   10. changing misconceptions about eating and weight
   11. correcting distorted body image
   12. changing family interactions
   13. in some families, parents abdicate authority and expect children to be very mature
   14. reframing the symptom and telling the family that the anorexic symptoms are voluntary
   15. weight restoration can be fast but complete recovery takes years
   16. adolescents recover better than older patients and females better than males

B. Treatments for Bulimia Nervosa
   1. psychodynamic and cognitive approaches are the most commonly used
   2. group therapy often used
   3. self-help support groups
   4. Overeaters Anonymous (OA) assumes it's a lifelong illness of food addiction
   5. behavioral therapy may include monitoring and keeping diary of eating behavior and emotions
   6. exposure and response prevention
   7. antidepressant medications can be helpful
   8. untreated, lasts for years but 40% show immediate response to treatment

V. Eating Disorders: The State of the Field

   A. Prevalence Increasing

   B. Various Factors and Personality Types Similar for Both Disorders

   C. Better Treatments Still Needed

   D. Patient-initiated National Organizations

Learning Objectives:
1. Explain the relationship between prevalence of eating disorders and thinness obsession.
2. Know at what age groups anorexia and bulimia are most common.
3. List the five central features of anorexia nervosa.
4. Compare and contrast the various behavioral patterns of anorexia and bulimia.
5. Explain why bulimics find purging behavior to be reinforcing.
6. Describe how eating disorders tend to be initiated.
7. Compare and contrast how bulimics and anorexics perceive their eating disorders.
8. Describe possible medical problems caused by eating disorders.
9. Explain how each of the following factors can place a person at risk for an eating disorder: sociocultural pressures, family environment, ego deficiencies and cognitive disturbances, biological factors, and mood disturbances.
10. Describe the enmeshed family pattern.
11. Explain the concept of weight set point.
12. Know the goals of treatments for eating disorders.
13. Describe treatments for anorexia nervosa.
14. Describe treatments for bulimia nervosa.
15. Discuss the success rate of eating disorders treatment.

Instruction Suggestions:
1. *Mini-Lecture.* **Twin Studies and Determining the Genetic Aspects of Weight**
   Do you think your weight is determined more by your ancestry or by your lifestyle? A 1990 study by Stunkard analyzed weight and height records from the well-known Swedish Adoption/Twin Study of Aging. Involving 247 identical twin pairs and 426 fraternal twin pairs, the study found that twin siblings ended up with similar body weights whether or not they were raised in the same home. The correlation in body-mass index for the identical twins reared apart was nearly the same as that of identical twins

reared together. Correlations with biological parents were higher than with their adopting parents. When both biological parents were obese, 80% of the offspring were also overweight. This study found that childhood environment did not strongly affect body weight.

In another study, Canadian researchers had twelve pairs of identical twins consume 1,000 extra calories a day for 84 days. Weight gains ranged from only nine pounds to nearly thirty pounds. Twin pairs tended to gain about the same amount of weight. Twin weight gains were more similar than to other nontwin siblings. In a May 1990 *New England Journal of Medicine* article, researcher Bouchard stated, "It seems genes have something to do with the amount you gain when you are overfed."

2. *Class Demonstration.* Try to find and use case studies of individuals who do not fit the pattern of having eating disorders in the adolescent years. Here are a couple of excerpts from former students that might be adaptable.

*P. started her eating disorder in her thirties, about the time her last child began going to school and her husband was busy at work. She simply started walking with friends and noticed she felt a lot better. Soon she walked much farther than they did, eventually walking a daily ritual all over city that she began as soon as the kids left for school and finished just minutes before they got home. She did the same walk even in snowy, below-zero weather or during thunderstorms. She denied herself food all day long and then after the family was asleep she would hitchhike to an all-night store, buy cookie ingredients and make them in an electric frying pan in the bathroom with the exhaust fan going so that her family wouldn't smell them. She would gobble down a double batch of soft cookies each night and then walk all day long the following day. Doctors had trouble diagnosing P.'s eating disorder because of her age.

*N. initially used her drinking problem to control her weight. She would drink so much she would vomit and that would keep her from gaining weight. When she became sober, she was very upset with her weight gain. In an eating disorders college class she learned about the behaviors of individuals with bulimia nervosa and started self-inducement of vomiting even though she was hearing all about the negative side effects of the pattern in her class. She finally had found a way of controlling her weight. Working through this pattern meant an intensive in-patient treatment program in her thirties; all the other patients were younger than eighteen.

*H. was a noted cook and had even had her picture taken with hundreds of cookbooks in the background when she was a featured cook in a regional newspaper. Yet, her obsession with good cooking was a way to deal with the preoccupation of food she had due to her self-starvation. She rarely tasted any of the great dishes she made. Within a year of being a featured cook, she died of medical complications of anorexia. She was in her thirties at the time of her death.

3. *Mini-Lecture.* **The Fat Mouse Research**
Researchers have bred a mouse that weighs ten times as much as a normal mouse. Not only does this mouse allow experiments that compare obesity with normal weight, it also allows experiments that compare differences between genetic overweight and overeating overweight.

The genetically fat mice have been found to be deficient in a protein made by fat cells (adipocytes). This protein adipsin is as much as ten times lower in genetically fat mice fed potato chips, candy bars, bologna, cookies, and marshmallows. It is speculated that adipsin may be a fat regulator for mice. As such, it circulates in the bloodstream and responds to changes in diet. For example, when food intake is restricted, adipsin levels rise. Current research includes injecting genetically fat mice with adipsin to see if weight decreases.

As yet, it is unknown whether human beings have an equivalent to adipsin. One area of research is complement factor D, which typically is used by the immune system to combat infections. This disease protector just might play a major role in regulating fat. 1985 research in the area of the fat-immune connection identified cachectin, a protein that causes emaciation in many cancer patients while actually fighting cancer.

4. *Class Activity*. Develop a list of cultural attitudes (and contractions) about food. Discuss these various values and how they might influence eating disorders.

5. *Class Project*. Assign students to analyze television ad messages about food. Have them contrast food ads on prime-time TV and children's TV shows. Is food sold as a biological necessity or as a reward, status object, and psychological need fulfiller ("You've got the right one, baby," "You deserve a break today," "We do it all for you.")?

6. *Small Group Discussion*. Have small groups of students discuss how food was used in their families. What messages did they get about food and eating? How and where was food used? Did families eat together? Were meal times pleasant? Was food punished? Was food seen as the enemy of fat? Have each group summarize what they discovered.

7. *Class Demonstration*. Emphasize the changes in ideal female body image by bringing in pictures of the ideals from various eras (a painting by Reubens, Lillian Russell, the delicate songbird of 200 pounds, Marilyn Monroe, the sex goddess who at 135 lbs. and only 5'5" would now be considered overweight, emaciated Twiggy of the '60s, and exercise guru Jane Fonda.

8. *Class Project*. Have students find examples of diet articles from popular magazines. Ideally find some very old ones. Analyze their advice quality and their emotional tone.

9. *Class Discussion*. Have students evaluate self-help groups like Overeaters Anonymous and various commercial enterprises such as Weight Watchers and NutriSystem. What do they have in common? What are their differences? What do they emphasize? How do students evaluate them?

10. *Class Discussion.* Discuss the relationship between food and emotions from different theoretical perspectives (i.e., psychodynamic, behavioral, biological, cultural).

11. *Lecture Additions.* Develop a brief lecture of what is known about good nutritional advice, such as low sugar, low fat, only a little meat, lots of fruits, vegetables, and grains, the value of fiber, the value of the vegetable group of cabbage, broccoli, and cauliflower.

12. *Class Activity.* Have students address the similarities and differences of eating disorders with each of the following mental disorders: obsessive compulsive, depression, drug addiction, phobic disorder, as well as codependency and workaholics.

13. *Class Discussion.* What assumptions do you make when you see a thin person? Fat person?

Topic Overview:
I. Substance Abuse and Dependence

   A. Drugs
      1. any substance other than food that changes bodily or mental functioning
      2. "drug" and "substance" used interchangeably

   B. Abnormal Functioning
      1. organic mental syndrome, a dysfunction of brain characterized by changes in behavior, emotion, or thought
      2. includes intoxication or hallucinosis

   C. Substance Use Disorder
      1. substance abuse is relying excessively and chronically on a drug so that it occupies a central position in one's life
      2. substance dependence is a physical addiction besides an abusing pattern
      3. tolerance refers to needing increasing doses to achieve the initial effect
      4. withdrawal symptoms are unpleasant, sometimes dangerous reactions that occur when drug users suddenly stop taking or reduce their dosage of a drug
      5. withdrawal symptoms can include muscle aches and cramps, anxiety attacks, sweating, nausea

   D. Prevalence
      1. 7% of all adults
      2. 37% have used an illegal substance at some time
      3. 48% of all high school seniors have used an illicit drug at least once
      4. 33% of high school seniors have used an illicit drug in the past year

II. Depressants

   A. Slow CNS Activity

   B. Alcohol
      1. two-thirds of the population drink alcohol
      2. 11% consume an ounce or more every day
      3. males outnumber females by two to one or as much as five to one
      4. ethyl alcohol rapidly absorbed into the blood through stomach and intestinal lining
      5. depresses or slows CNS functioning affecting judgment and inhibition, impairs fine motor control, increases light sensitivity, and then greater impairment

6. at 0.06% blood alcohol content, person is relaxed and comfortable, but by 0.09% person is intoxicated, and at 0.55% death would result (most pass out way before this level)
7. most alcohol is metabolized by the liver where the enzyme alcohol dehydrogenase converts it into acetaldehyde, which is then broken down into acetic acid and finally carbon dioxide and water
8. alcoholism affects 5-6% of all American adults currently and 13% at some time in their lives
9. alcohol abusers regularly drink excessively and feel unable to change their habit
10. one pattern is drinking large amounts of alcohol daily until intoxicated and therefore planning one's daily life around drinking
11. alcohol withdrawal delirium or delirium tremens (DT's) exhibited by alcohol dependent persons who stopped drinking in last three days
12. a rare withdrawal reaction is alcoholic hallucinosis, which features auditory hallucinations for as long as a few months
13. one of society's most dangerous drugs, destroying millions of lives, families, relationships, and careers, as well as being a factor in half of all suicides, homicides, assaults, rapes, and accidental deaths
14. a major problem among the young, with 5% of high school seniors drinking daily
15. cirrhosis, a scarred liver, is the ninth most frequent cause of death in the United States (28,000 deaths yearly)
16. also nutritional problems, which can lead to organic mental disorders: Wernicke's encephalopathy, Korsakoff's syndrome

C. Sedative-Hypnotic Drugs
1. in 1950s, the antianxiety drugs benzodiazepines (e.g., Valium, Xanax, Librium) were discovered
2. less impact on brain's respiratory center than barbiturates, therefore safer
3. however, high dosages can cause intoxication and an abuse or dependence pattern
4. 1% misuse anxiety drugs at some time
5. barbiturates can help tension and insomnia but they can be dangerously misused
6. low doses of barbiturates and benzodiazepines reduce excitement level by increasing synaptic activity of the inhibitory neurotransmitter GABA but achieve this differently, with only barbiturates affecting messages into the reticular formation
7. may prescribe for hypnotic effects and patients learn to use them to cope rather than to induce sleep and develop into an abuse pattern
8. tolerance develops rapidly
9. withdrawal symptoms include nausea, vomiting, weakness, malaise, anxiety, depression, and even barbiturate withdrawal delirium or amnestic disorder
10. lethal dosage remains the same even while body is building tolerance for its effects

D. Opioids
1. opium and drugs derived from it, e.g., heroin, morphine, codeine
2. morphine derived from opium in 1804 and used as a pain reliever and sleep aid (named for Morpheus, Greek god of sleep)

3. use increased during Civil War and morphine addiction became known as "soldiers' disease"
4. morphine was converted into a new pain reliever, heroin, in 1898, which mistakenly was believed to be non-addictive and turned out to be more addictive with more rapid tolerance
5. the various opioid drugs are called narcotics and they vary in potency, speed of action, and tolerance level
6. heroin is smoked, inhaled, injected beneath the skin and injected into the bloodstream
7. heroin injection brings on a short-lived rush followed by a several-hour pleasant, relaxed high or nod
8. heroin's effects are due to depressing the central nervous system and influencing endorphin receptor sites
9. in addition to pain relief, sedation, and mood effects, heroin causes nausea, pupil constriction, and constipation
10. withdrawal symptoms experienced right after the several-hour high beginning with anxious restlessness and a craving for heroin
11. in a few hours, there is profuse sweating, rapid breathing, and symptoms of a head cold with symptoms increasing for three days
12. heroin withdrawal distress peaks by the third day and gradually decreases over the next five days
13. daily habit can run over $200, so many support habit by theft and prostitution
14. most direct danger of heroin abuse is an overdose, which is most likely when a person resumes use after a period of abstaining
15. other risks are impure drugs and unclean needles leading to AIDS, hepatitis, and skin abscesses

III. Stimulants

A. General Description
1. act to increase activity of the central nervous system
2. increased blood pressure and heart rate and intensified behavioral activity, thought processes, and alertness

B. Cocaine
1. from the coca plant, the most powerful natural stimulant known, it has been processed into hydrochloride powder since 1865
2. only in the last few years have researchers realized how harmful cocaine is and how it produces its results
3. 24,000,000 Americans have tried cocaine, including 30% of all college students, and 6,000,000 use cocaine at least once a month
4. a euphoric rush of well-being and confidence along with feeling excited, talkative, and euphoric
5. as more is taken, stimulates other CNS centers and pulse increases, blood pressure rises, and breathing rate increases
6. cocaine intoxication involves poor muscle coordination, grandiose manner, poor judgment, and changeable temper
7. a severe state of intoxication, cocaine psychosis, involves confusion, anxiety, rambling, and incoherence

8. depressionlike letdown or "crashing," sometimes accompanied by headaches, dizziness, and fainting, which with low usage disappears in a day but with more use can lead to depression, deep sleep, or coma
9. cocaine abuse leads to feeling unable to stop using cocaine and poor social and work functioning with abstinence producing deep depression, intense fatigue, irritability, tremulousness, and anxiety
10. freebasing and injection create more abuse problems than snorting
11. cocaine dangers include depression and paranoia, overdosage due to effects on respiratory center, poor control of body temperature with inability to sweat, fatal heart problems

C. Amphetamines
  1. stimulant drugs made in a laboratory since the 1930s, including amphetamine (Benzedrine), dextroamphetamine (Dexedrine) and methamphetamine (Methedrine)
  2. used to try to lose weight, get athletic burst of energy, stay awake on the job, and induce more studying time, but not very effective at any of this
  3. pill, inject, free-basing
  4. low dosages increase energy and alertness and reduce appetite but in high dosages intoxication and psychosis and "crashing"
  5. quick tolerance
  6. as tolerance increases, may expend more energy than have and increase injuries and illness
  7. when regular abusers stop, deep depression and extended sleep

IV. Hallucinogens

A. Psychedelic Drugs
  1. "trips" that affect novel sensory experiences that can be exciting or frightening
  2. include LSD (lysergic acid diethylamide), mescaline, psilocybin, DOM, DMT, morning-glory seeds, kbufotenine, and PCP
  3. LSD developed by Hoffman in 1938 from the ergot alkaloids and experimented with by many in the 1960s
  4. hallucinogenic hallucinosis with intensified perceptions, particularly visual perceptions—distorting objects, breathing inanimate objects, geometric forms
  5. synesthesia, cross of the senses
  6. emotional changes from euphoria to depression, slowing of time
  7. physical symptoms: pupil dilation, sweating, palpitations, blurred vision, tremors, loss of coordination
  8. LSD affects neurons that use serotonin, which are involved in transmission of visual information and emotional experiences
  9. tolerance is minimal and no withdrawal symptoms but very potent and can develop hallucinogen delusional disorder or hallucinogen mood disorder
  10. about a quarter have flashbacks, sensory and emotional changes that unpredictably occur long after the LSD has left the body

B. Cannabis
  1. the hemp plant's (cannabis sativa) main active ingredient is tetrahydrocannabinol (THC) mainly in the resin of the leaves and flowering tops; the more THC, the more powerful the cannabis

2. varieties are collectively called cannabis—most powerful is hashish, intermediate is ganja, and weaker is marijuana
3. low doses produce feelings of inner joy and relaxation and either contemplative or talkative with a minority experiencing anxiety, paranoia, and apprehension and some noticing perceptual and time changes
4. physical changes: eyes reddened, faster heartbeat, appetite increase, dry mouth, drowsy, dizzy
5. high doses associated with visual distortions, body image alterations, hallucinations, confusion, panic, and impulsiveness

C. Marijuana Abuse and Dependence
   1. until 1970s, marijuana rarely led to pattern of abuse or dependence
   2. now used more frequently and with more potent marijuana—THC content of 10-15% compared to 1-5% in the 1960s
   3. chronic users have a tolerance and experience flulike withdrawal symptoms

D. Dangers of Marijuana
   1. occasionally panic reaction especially in people with emotional problems
   2. stronger marijuana means more impairment in complex sensorimotor tasks, e.g., driving
   3. interference with cognitive functioning, e.g., memory problems, concentration
   4. lung disease as one marijuana cigarette is equivalent to 16 tobacco ones in lung effects
   5. effects on human reproductive system
   6. mild and temporary suppressive effect on immune system
   7. incidence is starting to decline—4% of high school seniors smoke pot daily compared to 11% in 1978

V. Combinations of Substances

A. Cross-tolerance
   1. building up tolerance for one drug may build up tolerance for a similar drug although never used
   2. can use a similar drug to cut back on withdrawal symptoms from abused drug
   3. using antianxiety drugs, vitamins, and electrolytes during alcohol withdrawal to minimize delirium tremens

B. Synergistic Effects
   1. drugs used at same time may potentiate, or enhance, each other's effects
   2. by giving similar drugs such as alcohol, antianxiety drugs, barbiturates, and opioids
   3. other synergistic effects result when drugs have opposite or antagonistic actions

C. Polydrug Use
   1. carelessness or ignorance
   2. on purpose, especially among teenagers and young adults

VI. Explanations of Substance Abuse and Dependence

    A. The Genetic and Biological View
        1. twin, adoptee and animal studies suggest inherited predisposition
        2. alcoholics have livers that produce higher levels of acetaldehyde when
           metabolizing alcohol and have abnormal brain waves before or after drinking
        3. use may alter neurotransmitter activity, such as benzodiazepines lowering
           production of GABA or cocaine and amphetamines lowering production of
           dopamine and norepinephrine

    B. The Psychodynamic View
        1. dependency needs traceable to oral stage
        2. "substance-abuse personality"—dependent, antisocial, impulsive, depressive

    C. The Behavioral View
        1. reinforced by reduction of tension and sense of well-being
        2. Solomon's opponent-process theory

    D. The Sociocultural View
        1. dysfunctional families and family attitudes
        2. stressful regions of the country, e.g., higher rates of divorce associated with more
           alcoholism
        3. religious beliefs

VII. Treatments for Substance Disorder

    A. Insight Therapies
        1. address contributing psychological factors
        2. underlying conflicts and accepting feelings
        3. not highly effective

    B. Behavioral and Cognitive-Behavioral Therapies
        1. aversive conditioning
        2. covert sensitization
        3. teaching alternatives
        4. behavioral self-control training (BSCT) and relapse-prevention training

    C. Biological Treatments
        1. detoxification is systematic and medically supervised withdrawal
        2. either gradual decreases of drug or use of other drugs to reduce symptoms
        3. antagonist drugs to change effects of addictive drug
        4. drug maintenance therapy, such as methadone maintenance programs

    D. Self-Help Programs
        1. Alcoholics Anonymous has 650,000 members in 22,000 chapters
        2. peer support therapy

    E. Controlled Drug Use Versus Abstinence
        1. cognitive-behavioral theorists believe drinking can be retrained to be moderate
        2. AA says, "Once an alcoholic, always an alcoholic"
        3. both hard to achieve

VIII. Substance Use Disorders: The State of the Field

    A. Substance Use Still Rampant and Causing Many Problems

    B. New Drugs Keep Emerging

    C. Research Bringing Better Understanding

    D. Flourishing Self-Help Groups and Rehabilitation Programs

    E. Preventive Education

Learning Objectives:
1. Define the term drug.
2. Compare and contrast the terms substance abuse and substance dependence.
3. Explain the terms tolerance and withdrawal symptoms.
4. List commonly used depressants and explain their effects on the central nervous system.
5. Describe typical patterns of alcohol abuse and know the signs of physical dependence.
6. Discuss possible physical disorders caused by excessive alcohol intake.
7. Distinguish between antianxiety drugs and barbiturates and explain why barbiturate abuse is dangerous.
8. Know which drugs are opioids and be able to explain the effects of these narcotics on the brain.
9. Describe the typical physical, emotional, and behavioral effects of cocaine.
10. Describe the typical effects of amphetamine use.
11. Know the general effects of hallucinogens, such as hallucinogenic hallucinosis and synesthesia, as well as unpleasant effects, such as hallucinogen delusional disorder, hallucinogen mood disorder, and flashbacks.
12. Know the short-term and long-term effects of cannabis sativa use.
13. Explain cross-tolerance and a synergistic effect.
14. Discuss the biological view of substance misuse.
15. Explain the psychodynamic view of substance abuse.
16. Describe the behavioral view of substance abuse and how opponent process theory is used to explain the paradoxical effects of drugs.
17. Discuss the sociocultural view of substance abuse.
18. Compare and contrast insight theories and behavioral techniques in treatments for substance abuse.
19. Describe biological treatments of substance abuse and be able to define detoxification, antagonist drugs, and drug maintenance therapy.
20. Explain the role of self-help groups in combating substance abuse.

Instruction Suggestions:
1. *Class Discussion.* Discuss the need for drug searches and drug testing in the schools and workplaces. What is the balance between individual rights and resolving the "drug war"? Should your college conduct random drug testing for marijuana and cocaine? Arkansas has used blood tests, breathalyzer tests, and polygraph tests on high school students. New Jersey conducts spot searchers of lockers, gym bags, and purses, even though the Fourth Amendment outlaws spot searches.
2. *Class Activity.* Either orally or in written format, have students take the following quiz on

fetal alcohol syndrome, which Janet Simons put together in 1989 based on current magazine articles. Discuss the answers and whether they had a tendency to under- or overestimate FAS and their strategies for reducing the number of infants affected by FAS.

1. About _____ American babies are born each year with alcohol-related defects.
   A. 5,000
   B. 15,000
   C. 25,000
   D. 40,000
   E. 50,000

2. Of babies affected by alcohol, _____ are severely enough affected to be called FetalAlcohol Syndrome (FAS) babies.
   A. 2,000
   B. 6,500
   C. 12,500
   D. 18,000
   E. 25,000

3. FAS is responsible for _____% of all cases of mental retardation in this country.
   A. 5
   B. 10
   C. 15
   D. 20
   E. 35

4. Which group has the biggest risk for having a child with FAS?
   A. African-American
   B. Anglo-American
   C. Native American
   D. There are no differences in FAS rates among ethnic groups

5. Drinking during the first trimester does not lead to FAS.
   A. True
   B. False

6. Motor development can be impaired for breast-feeding babies whose mothers drink alcohol.
   A. True
   B. False

7. Some studies suggest that some injuries to the fetus from alcohol may be corrected in the womb if a mother gives up alcohol before her third trimester.
   A. True
   B. False

8. Barbiturates, opiates, and alcohol have similar effects on developing fetuses.
   A. True
   B. False

Answers to Fetal Alcohol Syndrome Quiz:
1. E   Actually, this is a conservative number.
2. C   Damage includes facial deformities, mental retardation, and heart abnormalities.
3. D   FAS is the primary threat to children's mental health, much greater than either
Down syndrome or spina bifida.
4. C   The risk for African-Americans is 6.7 times that of Anglo-Americans; for Native
Americans it is 33 times more likely than for Anglo-Americans.
5. B   Although risk may be minimal during the first two weeks, during the rest of the
first trimester the organs are developing and much damage can result.
6. A   Alcohol can be ingested in the breast milk.
7. A   Scandinavian, Boston, and Atlanta studies all indicate that some correction may
occur. At least size and healthiness improve, but there is no evidence that
intelligence is repaired.
8. B   Barbiturates and opiates affect the nervous system; alcohol can affect any cell.

3. *Class Discussion.* Do you think that pregnant women who use drugs should face criminal
prosecution? Do you think it would cut down on their drug abuse, or would it keep
women away from professionals providing prenatal care services because they might get
arrested? Is fetal abuse the equivalent of child abuse? Can you think of alternative
solutions to criminal charges? Since parents who smoke increase their young children's
risk for asthma, should smokers also be liable? Since cocaine use can lower sperm counts
for more than two years after stoppage, should wives be able to sue husbands for
infertility problems if the husband used to use cocaine? This is not just an abstract
discussion. In August 1989, 23-year-old Jennifer Johnson was found guilty of delivering
a controlled substance to a minor—her baby, who was born a cocaine addict. She could
have spent 30 years in prison but was sentenced to a one-year house arrest in a drug
rehabilitation center and 14 years of probation.

4. *Mini-Lecture.* **Athletes and Steroids**
What do you know about anabolic steroids? Some of you probably know someone who
has used steroids to improve their athletic skills. After all, between 6 and 15% of high
school boys have used or are using steroids. In college, about 5% of the athletes use
steroids. Anabolic steroids were the reason that Canadian track star Ben Johnson lost his
Olympic gold medal. Although our primary image of anabolic steroid usage is that of
athletes, the first major use of them was by Hitler's SS troops in World War II. They took
steroids to increase their aggressiveness levels. The first mention of athletic use was a
1954 report that Russian athletes were using anabolic steroids. Two years later American
athletes were choosing methandrostenolone, or Dianabol.

One technique used by athletes is the "stacking principle," or the simultaneous use of
different anabolic steroid preparations to saturate many receptor sites. A second
procedure is called the cycling method, and this procedure involves the cycling of
different steroids over a six- to twelve-week period in order to minimize negative effects
and to schedule specific drugs for different competition needs.

Why do athletes use anabolic steroids? They are used to increase strength, lean body
mass, and aggressiveness and to speed recovery from physical injury. However, usage

includes the following side effects: dramatic mood swings, sleep disturbance, male pattern baldness, acne, and altered libido. In males, there can be impotence, lowered sperm count, and gynecomastia (breast development). In females there can be masculinization, hirsutism (male pattern of body hair), and cliteromegaly (enlarged clitoris). Teenagers may experience precocious puberty. More serious side effects are possible: impeded growth, early heart attack or stroke, liver failure, liver cancer, and psychological addition.

Abnormal aggression, mood swings, and psychiatric dysfunctions also seem to increase with anabolic steroid use. A study of 41 steroid using football players and body builders found that 9 had affective syndrome and 5 had psychotic symptoms. In a separate study of health club members who used steroids, 90% reported episodes of aggressive and violent behavior.

5. *Lecture Additions.* You can add the following facts to your lecture on marijuana use and abuse.
*A 1987 study of employed persons between 20 and 40 years old found that 16% had used marijuana within the last month.
*A 1988 Baltimore study found detectable blood levels of marijuana in one-third of over a thousand patients treated for shock/trauma following accidents.
*Cannabis contains more than 400 chemicals, including 61 cannabinoids, 11 steroids, 20 nitrogenous compounds, 50 hydrocarbons, 103 terpenes, and benxopyrene. Little is known about how these various components affect the body.
*THC is fat soluble and binds tightly to blood proteins. This lets it be taken in by tissues well supplied with blood: ovaries, testes, liver, spleen, lungs, and kidneys.
*THC reaches the brain within 14 seconds of being smoked.
*THC may remain in body tissues for 30 days or more and be found in urine for a month after use.
*Medical consequences of high doses or chronic use are found for the pulmonary, central nervous, and reproductive systems. Possible complications: tachycardia, laryngitis, bronchitis, decreased REM sleep, panic attacks, paranoia, memory impairment, altered menstrual cycles, and lowered sperm count. Fetal organ development can be negatively altered. Marijuana use also makes it harder to learn new information.

6. *Lecture Additions.* Material that may be added to your lecture about cocaine:
*Cocaine bought on "the streets" has usually been "cut" (mixed) with other substances from 4 to 8 times. "Cuts" include mannitol, lactose, sucrose, caffeine, phenylpropanolamine, ephedrine, amphetamine, procaine, lidocaine, and benzocaine. "Cuts" add volume and allow bigger profits but increase medical risks.
*The street value of cocaine in 1986 was 6 times the price of gold.
*In the 1980s, cocaine-related strokes climbed, especially among adults in their twenties, and cocaine is now one of the leading causes of strokes in young adults.
*Other serious medical complications are: myocardial ischemia, hypertension, angina, hyperthermia, renal failure, and seizures. Seizures are more likely after intravenous or freebase cocaine use than with snorting.

7. *Class Activity.* This is a quiz designed by Lakeside Pharmaceutical that allows smokers to determine how dependent they are on nicotine. A score of 7 or higher indicates strong dependence. A answers receive no points, B answers receive 1 point, and C responses score 2 points.

1. How soon do you smoke after you wake up in the morning?
   A. after 30 minutes
   B. within 30 minutes

2. Do you find it hard to refrain from smoking in places where it's forbidden?
   A. no
   B. yes

3. Which of all the cigarettes you smoke in the day is the most satisfying?
   A. not the first
   B. first one in the morning

4. How many cigarettes a day do you smoke?
   A. 1 to 15
   B. 16 to 25
   C. 26 or more

5. Do you smoke more in the morning than during the rest of the day?
   A. no
   B. yes

6. Do you smoke when you are so ill that you're in bed most of the day?
   A. no
   B. yes

7. How high is the nicotine content of the brand you smoke?
   A. low
   B. medium
   C. high

8. How often do you inhale the smoke from your cigarettes?
   A. never
   B. sometimes
   C. always

8. *Class Demonstration.* Ask someone from Alcoholics Anonymous, Narcotics Anonymous, Overeaters Anonymous, or other self-help support groups for recovering substance abusers to visit your class. Ask the speaker to address the twelve steps, what typical meetings are like, and the general benefits of peer support. Other good speakers would be a worker in a detoxification treatment center or an in-patient treatment program.

9. *Class Activity.* Have students generate a list of possible ways to influence the numbers of persons who drink alcohol and develop alcoholism. After brainstorming as many ideas as possible, have students decide which aspects could be changed and have a large impact

on society. Possibilities include: changing the legal drinking age, education about dangers of alcohol with schoolchildren, noting the effects of strength and sweetness of available drinks (young people tend to drink wine coolers rather than scotch), images in TV and files (TV advertising that glorifies beer drinking or soap opera actors drinking alcohol rather than coffee).

10. *Lecture Additions.* Review material about the think-drink effect and add this to your lecture. Basically, subjects who thought they had a moderate amount of alcoholic drinks but instead had a tonic water drink made the behavioral changes associated with moderate drinking. Other subjects who had alcohol but thought they had none did not make these changes.

11. *Mini-Lecture.* **Classical Conditioning and "Needle Freaks"**
Most people hate needles. We hated getting shots at the doctor's office and we dread the thought of getting a needle injected into our jaw at the dentist office. How then do some individuals get to be "needle freaks"—persons who "love" their needle habit? Needle freaks use needles to shoot up their drug of choice, such as cocaine or heroin, but, if they have no drug, the "needle freak" might choose to shoot up some water just to be able to play with the needle. And, whether shooting up drugs or water, the needle freak doesn't hurry to get the needle part over—every aspect of getting ready to shoot is lovingly drawn out—slowed-down motion of tying a tourniquet around the arm, of filling the needle and making sure an air bubble will not be injected, and thumping the lower arm to help raise a much-used vein. For one of us to witness, the process would be agonizingly slow; for the "needle freak" each tiny detail is a building part of the high. The "needle freak" might even take a lot longer to find a usable vein than is needed because it heightens the anticipation of the rush.

The user's behavior can be explained with the classical conditioning model. Initially the drug (US) is what brings about the desired emotional effect (UR) and the needle is just a necessary vehicle. But, since the needle always precedes the drug, it begins to acquire pleasant associations with the added benefit of increasing the length of time that the desired emotion is experienced. Eventually, the needle (CS) itself is able to produce the pleasure (CR) even when water is injected rather than the drug. Can you come up with classical conditioning parallels for drinking alcohol and smoking pot?

12. *Class Discussion.* Discuss how drug use is portrayed in movies and television. Have there been any changes lately? You might be able to make a short videotape of some excerpts to aid the discussion. Many students will be able to offer examples, such as *Days of Wine and Roses, Arthur, Clean and Sober, The Lost Weekend, The Rose.*

13. *Class Demonstration.* Since some substance abusers receive criminal treatment rather than medical and psychological treatment, you might have a narcotics officer or a probation officer address this side of the issue. You can create a panel discussion by presenting those who treat versus those who punish during the same class period.

Topic Overview:
I. Sexual Dysfunctions

A. Introduction
1. problems in sexual functioning are very common
2. psychological effects include sexual frustration, guilt about failure, loss of self-esteem, emotional problems with sexual partner
3. most dysfunctions can be treated successfully in relatively brief therapy
4. apply to both heterosexual and homosexual couples

B. Types of Sexual Dysfunctions
1. DSM-III-R classifies according to phases of sexual response cycle described by Masters and Johnson with additions by Kaplan
2. can affect any of first three phases: desire, arousal, orgasm
3. no dysfunctions associated with resolution phase
4. associated with desire phase are hypoactive sexual desire, or lack of interest in sex, and sexual aversion, which is finding sex unpleasant
5. arousal phase marked by general physical arousal of increased heart rate, muscle tension, blood pressure, and respiration and pelvic vasocongestion leading to penile erection and swelled clitoris and labia and vaginal lubrication
6. arousal phase dysfunctions include: male erectile disorder (impotence) and female arousal disorder (frigidity)
7. the most common male sexual dysfunction in orgasm phase is premature ejaculation and much rarer is inhibited male orgasm
8. female disorder of orgasm phase is inhibited female orgasm
9. two other sexual dysfunctions are sexual pain disorders: vaginismus and dyspareunia
10. dysfunctions are described as lifelong ~~ ~~~ ~~~~~~ ~ ~~~ ~ ~~~~~~~~~~~~~~~

C. Prevalence of Sexual Dysfunctions
1. difficult to have accurate statistics
2. sex surveys typically have 25% refusal rates and participants are more liberal, experienced, and unconventional
3. hypoactive sexual desire is about 15% of males
4. only recently would a woman with a male partner who had hypoactive sexual desire suggest he needed therapy
5. erectile disorder occurs in about 8-10% of males and premature ejaculation is between 10-25%
6. majority of those with premature ejaculation are under 30 years
7. hypoactive sexual desire in 20-35% of females

97

8. 30-77% of women have orgasms, probably 50% fairly regularly and 20% of women occasionally have pain during intercourse and 1% have vaginismus

D. Causes of Sexual Dysfunctions
   1. influences of childhood learning, problematic attitudes and beliefs, biological causes, individual psychodynamic factors, and relationship issues
   2. hard to define hypoactive sexual desire—should be persistent, recurrent deficiency or absence of sexual fantasies and desire for sexual activity
   3. often those in therapy have virtually nonexistent sexual desire
   4. negative reactions in sexual aversion include panic attacks, nausea and vomiting
   5. sex drive can be affected by testosterone, luteinizing hormone, estrogen, and prolactin
   6. some prescription and illicit drugs can suppress sex drives, including drugs used to treat high blood pressure, ulcers, glaucoma, allergies, heart disease, convulsions, and mental disorders
   7. chronic physical illness can also suppress sex drive
   8. negative situations can cause hypoactive sexual drive
   9. affected by severely antisexual religion or culture
   10. being exaggeratedly hardworking and serious and viewing sex as frivolous or self-indulgent, being mildly obsessive-compulsive or being a homosexual in a heterosexual marriage
   11. being in an unhappy, conflicted relationship
   12. adopting culture's double standard, some men cannot feel sexual desire for a woman they love and respect or for a wife once the wife is also a mother
   13. effects of being molested or assaulted
   14. role of performance anxiety and the spectator role in both erectile failures and premature ejaculation
   15. as man ages, more intense, direct, and lengthy physical stimulation of penis may be needed for an erection
   16. inhibited ejaculation associated with neurological disease, multiple sclerosis, diabetes, and drugs that inhibit sympathetic arousal
   17. low arousal and inorgasmic women affected by cultural double standard, which demands that women suppress and deny their sexuality
   18. 50-75% of women molested as children or raped as adults have arousal and orgasm dysfunctions
   19. physiological conditions also affect women's arousal and orgasm as those with damage nervous system and interfere with arousal, vaginal lubrication, and orgasm; and medications can interfere with female orgasm
   20. vaginismus has no physiological cause and is a conditioned fear response
   21. dyspareunia usually has a physical cause such as injury during childbirth, undiagnosed vaginal infection, and endometriosis

E. Treatment of Sexual Dysfunctions
   1. in the 1950s and 1960s, behavioral therapists began to develop procedures
   2. anxiety-reduction approach was moderately successful but also needed was dealing with misinformation, negative attitude, and knowledge about techniques
   3. importance of Masters and Johnson's *Human Sexual Inadequacy* in 1970

4. first component is assessment and conceptualization of the problem with emphasis on principle of mutual responsibility
5. then providing accurate information about sexuality
6. then changing problematic attitudes, cognitions, and beliefs
7. eliminating performance anxiety and the spectator role through sensate focus and nondemand pleasuring
8. increasing communication and effectiveness of sexual technique
9. changing destructive lifestyles and marital interactions
10. four-element sequential treatment model for hypoactive drive and aversion: affectual awareness, insight phase, cognitive and emotional change, and behavioral interventions
11. for erectile failure, reducing performance anxiety, sensate focus with "tease technique," "stuffing technique"
12. with major physical problems, penile prosthesis, vacuum erection device, and vascular surgery
13. premature ejaculation treated with direct behavioral retraining procedures such as "stop-start" procedure and the "squeeze" procedure
14. inhibited male orgasm treated by reducing performance anxiety and ensuring adequate stimulation
15. female arousal and orgasm dysfunction techniques include self-exploration, body awareness, and directed masturbation training
16. vaginismic patients practice contracting and relaxing pubococcygeal muscle

II. Paraphilias

A. Introduction
1. recurrent and intense sexual urges and sexually arousing fantasies involving nonhuman objects, children, nonconsenting adults, or suffering and humiliation
2. only if repeatedly act on these urges or feel extreme guilt and shame
3. only deviant if with nonconsensual individuals or if used exclusively

B. Fetishism
1. use of an inanimate object or body part for sexual arousal exclusively
2. begins in adolescence
3. some commit petty thievery to get their objects or collect photographs of objects
4. fetishes as defense mechanisms
5. use of aversion therapy, covert sensitization

C. Transvestic Fetishism
1. transvestism or cross-dressing to achieve sexual arousal
2. heterosexual males

D. Pedophilia
1. sexual gratification with children
2. 4% 3 years or younger, 18% 4-7 and 40% 8-11 years; victim knows molester most of the time and sometimes incestuous; victims are girls or boys
3. usually develops in adolescence
4. most married and have other sexual difficulties and life frustrations
5. often alcohol abuse

6. immaturity as a primary cause
7. prison, aversion therapy, orgasmic reorientation

E. Exhibitionism
1. sexually arousing fantasies of exposing genitals to another to produce shock
2. more intense when under stress or having free time
3. majority married but most have unsatisfactory sexual relationships
4. aversion therapy, covert sensitization, arousal reorientation, social skills training, psychodynamic intervention

F. Voyeurism
1. recurrent and intense desires to observe people secretly as they undress or have sex
2. may masturbate while watching or fantasizing
3. usually begins before the age of 15 and tends to be chronic
4. a way to exercise power over others, possibly due to inadequacy or social inhibition
5. psychodynamic view of reducing castration anxiety

G. Frotteurism
1. recurrent and intense sexual urges about touching and rubbing against a nonconsenting person
2. fantasizes that it is a caring relationship
3. adolescence or earlier and less after the age of 25

H. Sexual Masochism
1. sexual urges to be humiliated, beaten, bound, or otherwise made to suffer
2. in relationships or in masturbation
3. masochistic sexual fantasies beginning in childhood and then acted out in adulthood
4. developed through classical conditioning

I. Sexual Sadism
1. sexually aroused by idea or doing infliction of physical or psychological suffering
2. fantasize about having total control over another
3. association between inflicting pain and being sexually aroused
4. modeling, underlying feelings of sexual inadequacy

J. Final Thoughts
1. affected by cultural norms
2. criteria of who is being hurt
3. homosexuality used to be considered paraphilia and that judgment affected laws and justified prejudice

III. Sexual Disorders: The State of the Field

A. Recent Understanding of Cause and Treatment of Sexual Dysfunctions

B. Less Advanced with Paraphilias

C. Much Research

D. Good Success Treating Sexual Dysfunctions

E. Need for Proper Education

Learning Objectives:
1. Distinguish between sexual dysfunctions and paraphilias.
2. Be able to describe each of the four phases of the sexual response cycle: desire, arousal, orgasm, and resolution.
3. Explain the two most common dysfunctions of the desire phase: hypoactive sexual desire and sexual aversion.
4. Describe the dysfunctions of the arousal phase: male erectile disorder and female arousal disorder.
5. Discuss the orgasmic sexual dysfunctions of premature ejaculation and inhibited male or female orgasm.
6. Define vaginismus and dyspareunia.
7. Describe the incidence of sexual dysfunctions in men and women.
8. Explain the role of sex hormones in sexual desire and activity.
9. Discuss how drugs and medications affect sexuality.
10. Know the possible etiologies of erectile failure and how diagnosis is made.
11. Discuss the etiology of premature ejaculation, female arousal and orgasmic dysfunctions, vaginismus, and dyspareunia.
12. Describe and evaluate typical sex therapy techniques.
13. Define paraphilias and fetishism and describe behavioral treatment.
14. Define transvestism, pedophilia, exhibitionism, voyeurism, and frotteurism.
15. Compare and contrast sexual masochism and sexual sadism.

Instruction Suggestions:
1. *Class Demonstration.* Bring in an assortment of respected sex therapy manuals to show to the class and discuss. You might want to find some old sex education books and address some of the outmoded information.

2. *Class Discussion.* Have the class (possibly in small groups) discuss what aspects of sexuality should be criminal acts. How would they define these crimes and what would the punishment be? Have them address sexual orientation issues (homosexuality, bisexuality), nonconsenting partners (children, relatives, rape, voyeurism, exhibitionism, date rape), and other topics brought up in the book. You might bring in well-known and highly publicized incidents such as Pee Wee Herman's arrest for masturbating in an adult movie theater.

3. *Class Demonstration.* Have a speaker from Planned Parenthood or a sex therapist address some of the common issues in sexuality.

4. *Lecture Additions.* You can point out how cultural norms, beliefs, and values influence what is considered healthy sexuality by pointing out historical terms such as nymphomaniacs (which in the Victorian era might be any woman who was regularly orgasmic and enjoyed sex) and masturbatory insanity. Point out that into the 1930s it was a medical belief that masturbation could cause fatigue, physical illness, and mental illness. These beliefs contributed to children being punished for "playing with themselves" and parents telling children such things as "If you play with that it will fall off," "If you do that your eyes will stay cross-eyed," and so forth.

5. *Class Discussion.* Discuss the concept of whether sexual orientation could be classically conditioned after presenting some of Storms' ideas. In general, research has shown that objects that are repeatedly paired with erotic stimuli come to acquire arousing properties on their own. In a 1981 article in *Psychological Review*, Storms suggested that classical conditioning determines one's erotic orientation. The initial US-UR connection is between masturbation (US) and pleasurable arousal (UR). Any fantasized images or tangible stimuli that are repeatedly paired with initial masturbatory experiences influence sexual orientation. Storms suggests that early sexual maturation and early masturbation would be associated with a homosexual orientation because under these circumstances the classical conditioning would occur at an age before heterosexual activities usually develop. Supporting his view, Storms suggests that homosexuals have more same-gender siblings than do heterosexuals and also that more college athletes experience early sexual maturation and college athletes have a higher incidence of homosexuality than other college students.

How convincing are Storms' ideas? What do you like and dislike about his explanation of sexual orientation? Can you think of information that would be inconsistent with his viewpoint? How would you conduct research on his hypothesis? If his model were correct, would sexual orientation be modifiable? How? Does his model suggest that families could learn how to control the sexual orientation of their children? What problems might result from trying to modify or control the development of sexual orientation? In view of societal changes, including sexuality in the media, if Storms is correct, would you expect the incidence of homosexuality to change? Why? Does classical conditioning explain the development of some of the paraphilias better than it does sexual orientation?

6. *Mini-Lecture.* **Sexual Addiction**
Working with a model similar to that of substance abuse, Patrick Carnes has described a four-step sexual addiction cycle. As a person's sexual addiction progresses through the four-step cycle, the addiction intensifies with each repetition. The first step is preoccupation, or the addict's mood and mindset being completely engrossed with thoughts of sex. The addict's mind state leads to an obsessive search for sexual stimulation. In the second step, the addict engages in rituals that move the addict toward sexual behavior. These special rituals serve to intensify the preoccupation and to add to the sexual arousal and excitement. The third step is the compulsive sexual behavior itself. The sexual addict is unable to stop this sexual act, which represents the culmination of the preoccupation and ritualization. The final step is despair, or the addict's total sense of hopelessness and powerlessness over the cycle.

Carnes suggests that the sexual addict has four central or core beliefs: (1) I am basically a bad, unworthy person; (2) No one would love me as I am; (3) My needs are never going to be met if I have to depend on others; and (4) Sex is my most important need.

Finally, there are four main signs of compulsive sexuality. First, the compulsive sexuality is secretive. The sexuality is abusive to the addict and others by being degrading, exploitive, or harmful. Third, sexuality is used to avoid painful feelings or it is the source of painful feelings. Fourth, compulsive sexuality is empty of a caring, committed relationship. Patrick Carnes has published material appropriate for both professionals and nonprofessionals who want to learn more about sexual addiction.

7. *Small Group Discussion.* Have the class generate a list of childhood sexual messages and misconceptions. Have class members evaluate common errors, prohibitions, and how these early beliefs have affected their lives.

8. *Class Discussion.* Why are there only male transvestites? Why aren't homosexual drag queens considered transvestites? Are there women who dress in male clothes for sexual gratification?

9. *Class Discussion.* Have the students decide what the criteria for exhibitionism are? Are career-minded nude dancers and strippers exhibitionists? Are their customers voyeurs? Are nudists exhibitionists? Are sculptors and artists who create nudes symbolic exhibitionists? Are some of the rock stars with fairly explicit videos exhibitionists? Are "dirty jokes" funny because of their exhibitionistic/voyeuristic satisfactions?

10. *Mini-Lecture.* **Healing After Child Sexual Abuse**
In her book *Healing Your Sexual Self,* Janet Woititz describes several of the coping mechanisms that victims of sexual abuse often use—resistance, lack of resistance (a compliance of body but not of spirit in a situation without escape), emotional shutdown, dissociative behavior, amnesia, blocking out the experience, identifying with others, and returning memories. Painful as it is, gaining in awareness of what happened seems to be the key to resolution.

The impact of childhood sexual abuse on childhood can include the following: a sense of being damaged, low self-esteem, guilt and shame, fear and lack of trust, depression and anger, confused role boundaries ("parentified"), uneven child development (or no childhood), and a sense of powerlessness. All of these experiences can become more generalized in adulthood if sufficient help is not available. In addition, there may be compulsive behavior, post-traumatic stress disorder, and unhealthy intimate relationships. It does not cause homosexuality; some adult heterosexuals and some adult homosexuals were sexually abused as children. It does contribute to compulsive overeating, anorexia nervosa, bulimia, self-mutilation, substance abuse, sexual addiction, and co-dependency, but all of these disorders can have other causative factors.

103

Woititz believes that the following are initial steps involved in sexual healing: (1) express what happened; (2) admit that life is unmanageable; (3) admit to being victimized and to needing help.

If someone else shares their sexual abuse (or other childhood abuse) with you, the following are helpful ways to respond, according to J. Patrick Gannon: (1) believe what you are told about the abuse; (2) accept what the person says are the consequences of having been abused; (3) reinforce that the abuse was the parents' responsibility; (4) accept the person's feelings about the family members; (5) provide empathy, support, compassion, encouragement, and hope; (6) encourage attempts to get good help.

Topic Overview:
I. Schizophrenic Statistics and Facts

A. Prevalence
1. one in a hundred persons worldwide
2. equal numbers of men and women diagnosed
3. two million Americans have been or will be diagnosed

B. Cost
1. financial cost is between $10 and $20 billion annually
2. great emotional impact on families
3. associated with suicide risk and physical illness

C. Risk Factors
1. more in lower socioeconomic classes
2. effects of stress of poverty
3. inability to maintain a higher socioeconomic class

D. Historically
1. condition once referred to as "madness"
2. in Bible, King Saul had the symptoms and David feigned it to escape enemies
3. Hippocrates thought etiology was an imbalance of body's humors
4. Galen first to call it dementia and blamed it on coldness and excess humidity in the brain
5. in 1865, Morel used the term demence precoce indicating an early and serious intellectual and mental deterioration
6. in 1899, Emil Kraepelin used dementia praecox
7. in 1911, Eugen Bleuler used schizophrenia as meaning "split within the mind"
8. Bleuler saw the main aspects of schizophrenia: (1) fragmentation of thought processes; (2) a split between thoughts and emotions; (3) a withdrawal from reality
9. Bleuler also correctly noticed that intellectual deterioration was not inevitable and many stabilized and even improved

II. The Clinical Picture of Schizophrenia

A. Symptoms of Schizophrenia
1. delusions, or illogical, absurd ideas strongly held
2. most common delusions: persecution, reference, grandiosity, and control
3. delusions of thought withdrawal
4. thought broadcasting
5. delusions of thought insertion

6. less common delusions include somatic and religious delusions
7. formal thought disorders are disturbances in the production and organization of thought
8. most common formal thought disorder is loose associations, or the rapid shifting from one topic to another in inconsequential and incoherent statements while believing that sense is being made
9. statements of total gibberish can be called word salad
10. neologisms are made-up words that have meaning only to the person using them
11. perseverating is repeating words and statements, clang is rhyming statements, and blocking is when thoughts seem to disappear from memory
12. some degree of disordered thinking may appear long before a full pattern of schizophrenic symptoms
13. a heightened sensitivity to sounds and sights and feeling flooded
14. others experience sensory blunting
15. hallucinations are perceptions in the absence of external stimuli and auditory hallucinations are most common
16. can occur in other senses too: tactile, somatic, visual, gustatory, olfactory hallucinations
17. hallucinations and delusional ideas often go hand in hand
18. many experience blunted affect or even flat affect
19. others have inappropriate affect
20. a disturbed sense of self—a question of "Am I?"
21. may withdraw emotionally and socially and become totally preoccupied with their own ideas and fantasies
22. 75% are less knowledgeable about everyday social issues than those with other psychological disorders
23. changes in volition and feeling drained of energy, disinterested in normal goals, and indecisive
24. loss of spontaneity in movement and development of odd grimaces, gestures, and mannerisms
25. catatonic stupor, catatonic rigidity, catatonic posturing, waxy flexibility, catatonic excitement are extreme psychomotor symptoms

B. The Course of Schizophrenia
1. prodromal phase in which symptoms are not yet prominent but there is deteriorating functioning and some social withdrawal and acquisition of peculiar habits and communication difficulties
2. active phase in which symptoms become prominent—sometimes triggered by stress
3. residual phase is marked by a return to the prodromal level of functioning
4. phases can last days to years and recovery may be complete but the majority have at least some residual impairment
5. best recovery when there was good premorbid functioning, precipitation by stress, abrupt onset, and late onset

C. Diagnosing Schizophrenia
1. used to be the "wastebasket category," and in the 1950s it was "Even a trace of schizophrenia is schizophrenia"
2. current criteria: at least 6 months, deterioration of functioning, not due to physical disorders, different from mood disorders

106

3. disorganized schizophrenia features confusion, incoherence, fragmentary delusions, fragmentary hallucinations, grimaces, odd mannerisms, flat and inappropriate affect, and "silliness"
4. catatonic schizophrenia features psychomotor disturbances and is helped by antipsychotic drugs
5. most prominent symptom of paranoid schizophrenia is organized system of delusions and hallucinations that guide the person's life, especially delusions of persecution and grandeur and this type can show much improvement
6. undifferentiated type is anyone who does not fit nicely into one of the categories
7. residual type if symptoms are now less intense but still present
8. acute cases had sudden onset, good premorbid functioning, affective symptoms, and good response to treatment and were more likely to be severe mood disorders
9. Type I schizophrenia are those dominated by positive symptoms (delusions, hallucinations, formal thought disorder) and Type II by negative symptoms (deficits)
10. Type I has better response to antipsychotic drugs
11. Type I linked to biochemical abnormalities and Type II associated to structural abnormalities

III. Views on Schizophrenia

A. The sociocultural View
1. many features of schizophrenia are caused by the diagnosis itself
2. a self-fulfilling prophecy
3. Rosenhan's study of pseudopatients
4. a minority suggest that schizophrenia is largely the creation of society
5. most societies have a category equivalent to schizophrenia, e.g., "nuthkavihak," and "were"

B. Genetic and Biological Views
1. inheriting a biological predisposition in accordance with a diathesis-stress model
2. schizophrenia is more common among relatives of schizophrenics than among relatives of nonschizophrenic people
3. 1% of general population but 10% of first-order relatives
4. identical twins have a higher concordance rate than fraternal twins
5. supported also by adoption studies
6. chromosomal mapping research using a technique called restriction fragment-length polymorphism
7. the dopamine hypothesis with evidence from phenothiazine effectiveness, Parkinsonian symptoms, amphetamine psychosis, and dopamine receptor sites
8. overactive norepinephrine or serotonin may be involved, but not as much as dopamine
9. autopsied brains of many schizophrenic people contain more dopamine receptors than those of nonschizophrenic people
10. one version suggests that viruses affect antibodies to stimulate dopamine receptors
11. Type II associated with enlarged ventricles, also some with smaller frontal lobes, cerebrums, craniums, lower density of neurons, and reduced blood flow

C. Psychological Views
1. regression to a pre-ego stage and make efforts to reestablish ego control
2. primary narcissism in which only their own needs are felt
3. primitive logic, or paleologic thought
4. operant conditioning
5. environmental reinforcements help produce and maintain schizophrenic behavior
6. Frieda Fromm-Reichmann's schizophrenogenic mother as cold, domineering, and impervious to the needs of others
7. research shows more mothers are shy, inadequate, withdrawn, anxious, suspicious, incoherent
8. double-bind messages
9. marital schism and marital skew
10. precipitation by stressful family situation
11. parents as displaying more conflict, more difficult communication, and more critical of and overinvolved with children
12. Laing believed schizophrenia to be a constructive process in which people try to cure themselves of the confusion and unhappiness caused by their social and family environment
13. initial symptoms lead to trying to clarify what is happening and the development of beliefs that fit the symptoms

IV. Schizophrenia: The State of the Field

A. Antipsychotic Drugs

B. Learning about Nature and Course of Schizophrenia

C. Different Types May Be Different Disorders

D. Caused by Combination of Factors

E. Studying Chromosome Markers, Brain Chemistry, and Brain Structure

Learning Objectives:
1. Define psychosis.
2. List and describe the primary symptoms of schizophrenia.
3. Know the prevalence of schizophrenia and when it typically appears.
4. Compare and contrast the prodromal phase, active phase, and residual phase.
5. Distinguish among the five categories of schizophrenia: disorganized type, catatonic type, paranoid type, undifferentiated type, residual type.
6. Compare and contrast Type I and Type II schizophrenia.
7. Describe the effects of being labeled schizophrenic, including the results of Rosenhan's influential study.
8. Discuss and evaluate the evidence that people inherit a biological predisposition to schizophrenia.
9. Discuss and evaluate the evidence that biochemical abnormalities and abnormal brain structures are the cause of schizophrenia.
10. Explain the psychodynamic view of schizophrenia.
11. Explain the behavioral view of schizophrenia.

12. Define the terms schizophrenic mother, double-bind communications, marital schism, and marital skew.
13. Explain and evaluate Laing's theory that schizophrenia is a constructive process.
14. Describe and evaluate the cognitive view of how persons with schizophrenia explain biologically induced hallucinations.

Instruction Suggestions:
1. *Lecture Additions.* You can use the historical information about schizophrenia to make the following points in your lecture: (1) schizophrenia was established as a mental disorder a long time ago; (2) traditionally, professionals have learned to make correct diagnoses before any effective treatment is available; and (3) workable treatments often have preceded the understanding of etiology.

2. *Lecture Additions.* When discussing Bleuler's views, you might compare the "split within the mind" definition with one schizophrenic's description of his experience as "like agitated bits of hamburger distributed throughout the universe" and when noting that Bleuler felt many with schizophrenia stabilized or even improved. Mention that for many years the standard was 1/3, 1/3, 1/3— 1/3 got well, 1/3 got better, and 1/3 couldn't be helped. Now, however, the last group has dropped to about 1/10.

3. *Class Activity.* Locate the Magic Ideation Scale in Eckblad, M. & Chapman, L.J. 1983. Magical ideation as an indicator of schizotypy. *Journal of Consulting and Clinical Psychology, 51*, 216-217. Use it here or in the personality disorders chapter. You can also present a few items from the Sc scale of MMPI.

4. *Class Discussion.* Have a discussion comparing New Age beliefs and experiences with those of schizophrenia. Look at channeling, auras, and astral projections in terms of both.

5. *Lecture Additions.* In discussing thought broadcasting, Jan Larson of the Menninger Foundation has talked about a man who had schizophrenia for many years and she was the first to tell him what thought broadcasting meant. He said, "You mean all along nobody has been able to hear my thoughts—that's just part of that schizophrenia?" Larson affirmed that to him and then asked him how believing that all his thoughts could be heard by others affected him. He replied, "Well, it sure makes for charitable thoughts."

6. *Class Discussion.* Have students propose reasons for why there are so many "contradictory symptoms" in schizophrenia, e.g., sensory flooding vs. sensory blunting, loose associations vs. blocking, flat affect vs. inappropriate affect, catatonic excitement vs. catatonic stupor, thought broadcasting vs. thought insertion.

7. *Class Activity.* Have students learn about schizophrenia by playing a Jeopardy-like game. You can use these categories and answers and have teams come up with appropriate answers.
DELUSIONS: persecution, somatic, thought broadcasting, thought withdrawal, thought insertion, reference
THOUGHT SYMPTOMS: loose associations, neologisms, word salad, clang association, blocking
OTHER SYMPTOMS: hallucinations, inappropriate affect, flat affect, catatonic stupor, waxy flexibility
TYPES: paranoid, catatonic, disorganized, undifferentiated, residual
EXPLANATIONS: inherited, dopamine hypothesis, double bind, marital schism, paleologic thought

8. *Class Activity.* Have groups of students develop scenarios of a schizophrenic with hallucinations developing delusions to fit. Share the examples with the whole class.

9. *Class Discussion.* Have students discuss their own occasional experiences with schizophreniclike symptoms, such as inappropriate affect (e.g., giggling during a sermon). What's the difference between their experiences and those of persons with schizophrenia? Also, share experiences of supposedly schizophrenic-creating behaviors, such as double-bind communications.

10. *Class Demonstration.* Appropriate speakers on aspects of schizophrenia include a psychiatrist, a group home worker, a NAMI advocate, a person with schizophrenia or a family member.

11. *Class Discussion.* The book mentions that schizophrenia was once a "wastebasket category." Have students discuss what might be today's "wastebasket categories." Possibilities include adjustment disorders, post-traumatic stress disorder, borderline personality disorder, multiple personality disorder, co-dependency, addictive personality.

12. *Class Activity.* In small groups, have students write patient descriptions of each type of schizophrenia and then have other groups try to guess the appropriate diagnosis.

13. *Class Activity.* Create a list of schizophrenic symptoms and read them to the class, having students quickly respond by raising right hand if a Type I symptom (positive) and left hand if Type II (negative). Which ones were easy (good agreement) and which ones were hard?

Topic Overview:
I. Institutionalization

   A. Past Institutional Care
     1. in 1793 Philippe Pinel made radical changes in treating imprisoned mentally ill and began moral treatment
     2. Pinel's humanitarian ideas spread throughout Europe and United States and large hospitals rather than asylums built
     3. new hospitals located in isolated, inexpensive areas did have goal of being a haven from stress
     4. by the mid-19th century, state hospital system overcrowded and underfunded and staff had limited knowledge and experience
     5. between 1845 and 1955 about 300 state hospitals established in United States and number of hospitalized patients increased from 2,000 to nearly 600,000
     6. shift from humanitarian care to order-keeping and efficiency
     7. disruptive patients physically restrained, isolated, punished
     8. if did not soon improve, sent to "back wards" and were warehoused
     9. treatments included hydrotherapy and lobotomy
    10. many additional symptoms developed under these conditions
    11. social breakdown syndrome: extreme withdrawal, anger, physical aggressiveness, loss of interest in personal appearance and functioning

   B. Improved Institutional Care
     1. milieu therapy is changing institutional environment so that patients can have meaningful activity, responsibility, and self-development
     2. originated by Maxwell Jones in 1953 to have a residents' community engaged in establishing rules and determining sanctions and developing schedules
     3. superior to custodial care and sometimes improvement enough to leave hospital
     4. in many forms from better interpersonal interactions to meaningful work activities
     5. token economy programs as systematic application of operant techniques to alter dysfunctional behavioral patterns
     6. first token economy established by Ayllon and Azrin at Illinois hospital and involved tokens being redeemed for privacy, privileges, staff interactions, religious activities, recreation, and shopping
     7. token economy programs need specificity, flexible reinforcements, response costs, and staff participation
     8. some token economy programs operant as leveled programs, with different levels of difficulty

9. to help generalize to nonhospital setting, token economies need to become partial reinforcement schedules, use social reinforcements, and include a fading process

II. Antipsychotic Drugs

A. History
1. discovered in 1950s and produced a treatment revolution
2. eliminate many symptoms and are almost always part of treatment
3. in 1940s, medical researchers found certain drugs that blocked release of histamine and helped with hay fever—a group called phenothiazines
4. use of these drugs by Laborit to try to prevent anesthetized patients from experiencing a sudden drop in blood pressure and going into shock
5. phenothiazines did not affect blood pressure but did calm patients before surgery, especially chlorpromazine

B. Modern Neuroleptic Drugs
1. in 1954, chlorpromazine (Thorazine) marketed in the United States as an antipsychotic medicine
2. neuroleptic drugs often produce effects similar to symptoms of neurological diseases
3. phenothiazine group includes chlorpromazine (Thorazine), thioridazine (Mellaril), mesoridazine (Serentil), fluphenazine (Proxlixin), and trifluoperazine (Stelazine)
4. other chemical classes include haloperidol (Haldol) and thiothixene (Navane)
5. apparently reduce schizophrenic symptoms by reducing excessive activity of dopamine
6. after taking for a while, the dopamine-receiving neurons apparently grow additional, but now normal, dopamine receptors

C. Effectiveness of Antipsychotic Drugs
1. research shows effectiveness for many patients
2. 50% rated as "normal" or "borderline normal" compared to only 15% of placebo group
3. drugs alone or those with drugs and psychodynamic therapy improved equally and least improved was only psychodynamic or only milieu therapy
4. schizophrenic symptoms typically return if drugs are stopped too soon
5. do best at alleviating positive symptoms than negative symptoms

D. Unwanted Effects of Antipsychotic Drugs
1. extrapyramidal effects because they are from the extrapyramidal areas that regulate motor activity
2. effects that resemble Parkinson's disease, e.g., severe and continuous muscle tremors, muscle rigidity, slow movement, shuffling, little facial expression
3. Parkinson's caused by underactive dopamine activity in the substantia nigra and that is where antipsychotic drugs block dopamine activity
4. in most cases, these unwanted effects can be reversed by an anti-Parkinsonian drug, e.g., benztropine (Cogentin) taken with the antipsychotic drug
5. dystonia is a condition of involuntary muscle contractions, causing bizarre and uncontrollable movements of the face, neck, tongue, and back

6. akathisia is a very high degree of restlessness and agitation with great discomfort in the limbs and is hard to control without reducing dosage of antipsychotic drugs
7. tardive dyskinesia may occur after being on antipsychotic drugs at least a year and symptoms include involuntary writhing or ticlike movements of the tongue, mouth, face, or whole body
8. may have single symptom of tongue flicking or be as severe as continual rocking
9. tardive dyskinesia occurs in 10-20% of those taking neuroleptic drugs for extended time periods, and especially by those over 55 years old
10. tardive dyskinesia can be difficult or impossible to eliminate
11. looking for newer antipsychotic drugs that may be effective with fewer side effects, and some believe clozapine is a step in that direction

III. Psychotherapy

A. History
1. psychotherapy not often useful before antipsychotic drugs
2. primary task is winning trust of schizophrenic and building close relationship
3. Frieda Fromm-Reichmann would tell clients that they could exclude her from their private world and hold on to their disorder as long as they wished
4. Harry Stack Sullivan thought therapy must be their most secure relationship ever and Otto Will emphasized total acceptance and love
5. effective drugs enable schizophrenics to examine themselves and make behavioral changes

B. Insight Therapy
1. experience a more important factor than orientation
2. successful therapists are more active, set limits, express opinions, and challenge patient statements

C. Social Therapy
1. practical advice and life adjustment
2. issues of self-management, problem solving, decision making, social skill development
3. group or individual therapy

D. Family Therapy
1. 25-40% of recovering schizophrenics live with parents, siblings, spouses, or children
2. higher relapse rate if with families that are emotionally expressive and demanding than if with cooler, detached relatives
3. family members have difficulty adjusting to schizophrenic's withdrawal
4. helping to deal with family pressures, good use of family resources, and limited problematic family interactions
5. family support groups

IV. The Community Approach

  A. History
    1. 1950s, Joint Commission on Mental Illness and Mental Health
    2. 1960, commission issued a report called *Action for Mental Health*
    3. recommended transfer of patients from state institutions to local hospitals and mental health clinics
    4. 1963, Congress passed the Community Mental Health Act
    5. deinstitutionalization
    6. about 600,000 institutionalized in 1955 and now under 125,000
    7. "revolving door" syndrome

  B. Effective Community Care
    1. communities with effective care have patients who make progress
    2. community mental health centers for medications, therapy, emergency care
    3. short-term hospitalization for diagnostic evaluation, observation, supervision, and precise monitoring of medications
    4. aftercare after a short hospitalization
    5. other needed facilities include day centers or day hospitals, halfway houses, sheltered workshops, and occupational training

  C. Inadequacies in Community Treatment
    1. in 1955 only 23% of all patients in treatment were in outpatient care and now it is 76%
    2. less than half of schizophrenics receiving appropriate community mental health services
    3. problems with poor coordination of services and shortage of services
    4. a great number of released schizophrenic patients become homeless with about a third of the homeless having a severe mental disorder

  D. The Promise of Community Treatment
    1. need to have better functioning
    2. National Alliance for the Mentally Ill
    3. National Mental Health Consumers Association
    4. worldwide movement toward community care

V. Treatments for Schizophrenia: The State of the Field

  A. From Nothing Effective to an Arsenal of Good Weapons

  B. Start with Outpatient Basis with Medications and Counseling/Support Services

  C. Combined Approach Increases Functioning

  D. Better Knowledge Through Research

  E. Need for Better Treatments

  F. Need to Deal with Societal Problems such as Homelessness

Learning Objectives:
1. Explain how treatment for schizophrenia has changed over the last fifty years.
2. Compare and contrast milieu therapy and token economy programs.
3. Discuss how neuroleptic drugs work and know which symptoms they alleviate.
4. Discuss the undesirable effects of neuroleptic drugs and how they are treated.
5. Evaluate the role of therapy in treatment of schizophrenia.
6. Explain deinstitutionalization and discuss its effect on community approaches.
7. Discuss problems associated with the community mental health movement, including the "revolving door" syndrome, poor coordination of services, and shortage of services.
8. Explain the relationship between schizophrenia and homelessness.
9. Discuss the role of national interest groups in community treatment for schizophrenics.

Instruction Suggestions:
1. *Lecture Additions.* When lecturing on milieu therapy, introduce the concept of *narrow therapeutic corridor.* According to this concept, each of us has a range of optimal stimulation—in terms of sensory input, emotional experience, and general activity. Too little, and individuals become bored or depressed. Too much, and individuals become stressed or inefficient. College students experience their own therapeutic corridor during the semester—when little is happening, they tend to feel underchallenged, lonely, bored, and depressed. However, at certain times of the semester (such as mid-terms, when termpapers are due, and final exam time) the level goes beyond the healthy corridor and students "freak out" with anxiety, irritability, and other negative experiences. For schizophrenics, the therapeutic corridor is more narrow and lower levels of activity are needed. Due to sensory overload and overactivity of dopamine receptors, what is a normal good level for nonschizophrenics is overwhelming for them and triggers symptoms. On the other hand, when hospitalized, so little may be happening that schizophrenics then have additional symptoms due to boredom. The key is for professionals and caring family members to help schizophrenic patients structure activities so that they fit into their narrow therapeutic corridor.

2. *Lecture Additions.* One of the ways in which behavioral therapists can help patients with schizophrenia is to teach them to come off as normal with the symptoms that remain while on good medication. Jan Larson of the Menninger Foundation tells of a patient whose primary symptom was feeling like his head was not attached to the rest of his body. The patient had coped with this unpleasant sensation and belief by wearing a tie up high on his neck. This odd appearance kept him from being hired for simple jobs that he would be able to manage. His therapist solved this problem by switching him to turtleneck sweaters. Other patients are taught to control their auditory hallucinations by devoting several minutes in the morning and evening to listening to what they have to say and the rest of the time having the voices fade into the background. On the few occasions that this strategy fails, patients are instructed to pick up a phone and dial an automated weather report and then speak to the voices so that it appears to others to be a normal telephone conversation.

3. *Class Demonstration.* Ask a social worker, halfway house worker, or psychiatrist to come and address their role in the treatment of schizophrenia.

4. *Mini-lecture.* **HEE and LEE Families and Training Families**
High expressed emotion (HEE) families have the following qualities: (1) they make frequent critical comments involving disapproval, resentment, dislike, or guilt induction; (2) personal criticism is used more than behavioral criticism; and (3) marked emotional overinvolvement as shown in overprotective attitudes, frequent intrusions, and constant worrying over small matters. HEE relatives often believe that the schizophrenic's bizarre behavior could be self-controlled.

Low expressed emotion (LEE) families are low-keyed, calm families who do not display HEE behaviors and tend to believe that schizophrenia is an illness and not a willful behavioral display.

When schizophrenic patients return to their families, expressed emotion style becomes the best single predictor of relapse (along with medical compliance). Patients in HEE homes have a 58% relapse rate and those from LEE homes have a 16% relapse rate. The good news is that HEE families can be taught LEE style and the result is a much lower relapse rate.

How should family members, friends, and others related to schizophrenic patients behave?
1. Communicate briefly, concisely, and clearly.
2. Do not make fun of delusions or try to talk the patient out of delusions, but ask the patient to express delusions only in private.
3. Expect the schizophrenic to be emotionally aloof and often to avoid conversations.
4. Provide a place where the person can withdraw and be alone.
5. Minimize noise and number of social events in the home.
6. Help the person establish a predictable, simple daily routine.
7. Help the person find leisure activities with low sensory input and usually without interpersonal interaction.
8. Develop a quiet, calm, confident attitude.

5. *Class Discussion.* Discuss some of the controversies around neuroleptic drugs. Check news magazines and papers for the latest controversies. One current controversy involves clozapine—how expensive blood tests to regulate this drug may have been overcontrolled and overexpensive.

6. *Class Discussion.* Who would like to work with schizophrenics? Of students wishing to be professional counselors, who has the goal of working with this mental disorder? Few, if any, will volunteer. Why? Some claim that counselors want YAVIS clients— young, attractive, verbal, intelligent, and social. Schizophrenic patients don't really fit this category. What would be the rewards of working with schizophrenic patients?

7. *Class Demonstration.* Have a speaker come from the National Association for the Mentally Ill or share some of their literature with your class.

Topic Overview:
I. Introduction

   A. Terms
      1. personality as unique, integrated pattern of behavior, perception, and emotion
      2. enduring consistencies are called personality traits
      3. personality disorders are inflexible, maladaptive personality traits that impair social or occupational functioning or cause intense distress
      4. personality disorders develop by adolescence and continue through adulthood

   B. Incidence
      1. about 10% of general adult population
      2. over half of those in treatment

   C. DSM-III-R Axes
      1. Axis I - vivid, discrete psychological problems
      2. Axis II - longer-standing forms of dysfunctioning beginning in childhood and persisting through adulthood
      3. if diagnosed on Axis I, then must also consider Axis II
      4. Axis I as extensions of Axis II personality disorders and personality disorders as extremes of normal personality traits
      5. personality patterns as best single predictors of mental disorders, responsiveness to therapy and drugs, and overall course of mental disorder

II. Models of Personality Disorders

   A. Three Major Clusters
      1. Cluster A - odd or eccentric, detached qualities (schizoid, paranoid, schizotypal)
      2. Cluster B - overly dramatic, reactive, emotional, erratic, intrinsically unstable, (antisocial, narcissistic, histrionic, borderline)
      3. Cluster C - pervasive anxiety, fearfulness, obsessiveness (dependent, passive-aggressive, obsessive compulsive, avoidant)

   B. Alternative Schema: Pervasive Reinforcements
      1. DSM-III-R clusters widely accepted but criticized for failing to consider underlying causal themes
      2. understanding types, sources, and instrumental processes of reinforcements that pervade one's life
      3. types of reinforcers are positive (enhancing, bringing pleasure) and negative (prevent or relieve psychological pain)

4. sources are self vs. others
5. instrumental processes can be active or passive

III. The Basic Personality Disorders

  A. Antisocial Personality Disorder
    1. 3% of men and 1% of women in the United States
    2. older names: psychopathy, sociopathy
    3. lifelong history of misconduct—as children playing truant, vandalizing, fighting, being cruel to animals and people
    4. as adults, no steady job, not meeting financial obligations, inadequate parenting, illegal activities
    5. indifference to others and can lie for gain or pleasure with little remorse
    6. among those with disorder, men are 5 times and females 10 times more likely than average to have biological relatives with the disorder
    7. reinforcement scheme: active, self-focused, positive
    8. neuronal hypersensitivity in the amygdala of the limbic system lowering the biological threshold for impulsive, aggressive, and egocentric behavior
    9. parental hostility and deficient parenting
    10. severe socioeconomic hardship
    11. suffered parental or societal abuse or neglect and overcompensates and is vindictive

  B. Narcissistic Personality Disorder
    1. Greek myth about Narcissus dying due to pining away longing for own reflection in a pond
    2. pervasive fantasies of success, beauty, or remarkable talent with extreme self-focus, so that they look to others only to further their own goals
    3. actually feel worthless, wounded by criticism, and envious
    4. driven to achieve but bogged down in depression and dysfunction
    5. reinforcement scheme: passive, self-focused, positive
    6. behavior patterns designed to extract praise, admiration, and special consideration
    7. narcissistic injury, when temporarily overwhelmed by personal failure or through rejection, but abates relatively rapidly
    8. excessive, unconditional parental valuation of the child with overindulgence and failure to set limits
    9. long-term therapy and social skills training

  C. Histrionic Personality Disorder
    1. live in dramatic emotionality and constant pursuit of attention and emotionally elaborate on even small events
    2. center stage by being charming, attractive, and seductive
    3. controlling in relationships, need constant praise and reassurance, and look for authority figures to solve all their problems
    4. reinforcement scheme: active, other-focused, negative
    5. parental pattern: minimal punishment, reinforced overly dramatic social performing, unusual or inconsistent positive reinforcement for socially acceptable behavior

D. Dependent Personality Disorder
1. rely on others even to make small decisions
2. more women than men
3. can't do any project alone, needy of praise, sensitive to rebuffs, fearful of losing relationships, demean themselves to please others, don't ask for their needs
4. reinforcement scheme: passive, other-focused, negative
5. inept self-image, behavioral incompetence, self-sacrifice
6. contributing factor may be deficient physical stature or health status
7. parental overprotection so don't develop competence
8. general feelings of unattractiveness or lack of intelligence
9. in counseling, encouraged to express their feelings, opinions, and preferences without fear of rejection and taught assertiveness
10. psychological growth and progression toward autonomy halted at level of adolescence

E. Passive-Aggressive Personality Disorder
1. seeking to control the lives of the people close to them by indirect means, including resenting and protesting reasonable requests, criticizing others, and being inefficient in tasks
2. reinforcement scheme: active, ambivalent, negative
3. characteristically cynical, skeptical, untrusting, pessimistic, misanthropic, sulky, moody, obstinate, and resentful
4. pronounced cyclical hormonal or neurotransmitter fluctuations
5. parental inconsistency
6. playing role of moderator in a conflicted family environment
7. modeling parents' passive-aggressiveness
8. in therapy, late for appointments, not paying bill, missing sessions, making excuses for not complying
9. social skills training and general assertiveness training

F. Obsessive Compulsive Personality Disorder
1. very intent on doing everything right but their extreme efforts impair their productivity and their relationships
2. perfectionists needing to meet such high standards that tasks remain unfinished because they can not be good enough
3. demand perfectionism from others and even plan their leisure time
4. viewed as emotionally cold and moralistic
5. mostly men
6. reinforcement scheme: passive, ambivalent, negative
7. at least one parent overcontrolling and unskilled at expressing love and affection or neglectful, abusing parents
8. taking on responsibility in a dysfunctional family and growing up too quickly
9. modeling
10. biological basis with serotonin involved
11. social skills training, relaxation training, encourage risk taking, cognitive techniques to gain cognitive flexibility
12. preference for highly structured, goal-oriented methods

G. Avoidant Personality Disorder
1. so fearful of being rejected that they give no one an opportunity to reject them, or to accept them
2. unable to establish the social ties for which they yearn
3. persons with social phobias fear specific social contexts, avoidant individuals fear relationships themselves
4. reinforcement scheme: active, negative, unable to obtain from self or others
5. biological factors, such as dysfunctioning in the brain's limbic system
6. hypersensitivity to stimulation may cause severe uncomfortableness with some interpersonal situations, e.g., parental or peer rejection
7. treatment to reduce anxiety (e.g., drugs, biofeedback) and desensitization to rejection
8. assertiveness training, social skills training, cognitive therapy

H. Schizoid Personality Disorder
1. do not yearn for close ties with anyone and avoid social contact because they genuinely prefer to be alone
2. lifelong indifference to other people with little pleasure being with relatives or friends
3. no interest in either sex or marriage
4. reinforcement scheme: passive, unable to obtain reinforcements from self or others, negative
5. biologically influenced involving dopamine
6. early childhood trauma, abuse, and neglect or fragmented pattern of family communication, very rigid home environment, and reinforced social isolation
7. in therapy establishing empathic relationship, acknowledge resistance to self-disclosure

IV. The Severe Personality Disorders

A. Paranoid Personality Disorder
1. shun close relationships because they trust no other
2. excessive trust in their own ideas and abilities
3. expecting to be hurt and deceived so reading the worst into others' behaviors
4. reinforcement scheme: active, self-focused, negative
5. an extension of either the antisocial, narcissistic, or obsessive compulsive personality disorder
6. paranoid-antisocial rooted in abusive or neglectful parental behavior
7. paranoid-narcissist rooted in parental overvaluation and the need for control
8. paranoid-compulsive rooted in persistent parental criticism and lack of parental approval
9. most likely to emerge when a person with one of the less severe disorders is faced with extreme stress at a critical developmental juncture
10. forming a therapeutic alliance by agreeing that the world is indeed a threatening place at certain times and in certain ways
11. helping to be more competent at discriminating real threats from perceived ones
12. tendency to threaten to sue may be an obstacle in therapy

B. Borderline Personality Disorder
   1. instability is the hallmark
   2. painfully uncertain of themselves, their image, sexual orientation, life goals, and values and complain of feeling "empty" or "bored"
   3. prone to depression, anxiety, anger, and impulsive behavior (e.g., binging, drinking, attempting suicide)
   4. marked by dysfunctions in relationships and marked instability of mood
   5. one of the most frequently diagnosed personality disorders
   6. extension of the histrionic, dependent, or passive-aggressive personality disorder
   7. reinforcement schedule: vacillating
   8. almost certainly linked to family dysfunction: parental neglect, parental inconsistency, contradictory parental communications, physical and emotional trauma
   9. during key developmental periods, dysfunctional families may cause dysfunction in the neurons within the limbic system
   10. remarkably resistant to treatment
   11. establish predictable boundaries, therapist takes active, supportive role, help in recognizing self-destructive, maladaptive aspects of behavior, help in identifying underlying needs and motives, monitor countertransference

C. Schizotypal Personality Disorder
   1. 3% of Americans have egocentric, dysfunctional symptoms that are milder than schizophrenia
   2. often believe that others are watching or talking about them, use magical thinking, have peculiar perceptions, are slovenly, talk to themselves, speak in a vague and rambling manner, and have blunted or inappropriate emotions
   3. an extension of avoidance and schizoid personality disorders
   4. reinforcement schemes: deficit in each area
   5. some suspect role of dopamine
   6. parental abuse, neglect, and psychological malnourishment
   7. milder variations may respond rather well to treatment

V. The Provisional Personality Disorders

A. Sadistic Personality Disorder
   1. active attempts to hurt and humiliate others, enthralled by violence and torture
   2. want to control and coerce others
   3. may embarrass children or subordinates by disciplining publicly and harshly
   4. may restrict others' freedom
   5. may hurt others with deliberate untruths
   6. often men who were abused as children or witnessed a parent being abused
   7. different than spouse abuse and sexual sadism
   8. reinforcement scheme: active, self-focused, positive
   9. perceptions of pain and pleasure are distorted so that pleasure is experienced by inflicting pain

B. Self-Defeating Personality Disorder
   1. habitually self-sacrificing, not engaging in pleasurable activities
   2. uncomfortable when things go well for them and experience guilt or depression at success

3. attracted to exciting but uncaring people
4. more women, many of whom were abused as children and many with deep depression
5. outdated label: masochistic personality disorder
6. martyrdom with self-effacing, servile behavior
7. reinforcement schedule: passive, others, negative

VI. Personality Disorders: The State of the Field

  A. Rebound in Popularity

  B. Difficulty in Identifying These Broad Problems

  C. Development of Unifying Principles and Themes

  D. Need for Research

Learning Objectives:
1. Define personality, personality traits, and personality disorders.
2. Compare and contrast the DSM-III-R clusters of personality disorders with the organization developed by Theodore Millon.
3. Describe the characteristics and etiology of antisocial personality disorder.
4. Describe the basic features of narcissistic personality disorder.
5. Describe the main characteristics of histrionic personality disorder.
6. List the primary characteristics of dependent personality disorders.
7. Describe the main features of passive-aggressive personality disorder.
8. Describe the characteristics of obsessive compulsive personality disorder.
9. Compare and contrast how those with avoidant personality disorder and those with schizoid personality disorder interact with people.
10. Describe the paranoid personality disorder and explain its possible etiology.
11. Explain the etiology of borderline personality disorder and describe its principle features.
12. Compare and contrast schizotypal personality disorder and schizophrenia.
13. Describe the two provisional personality disorders of aggressive (sadistic) personality disorder and self-defeating personality disorder.

Instruction Suggestions:
1. *Class Discussion.* Since this chapter deals with imbalanced personality patterns that develop early in life and last, it might be a good place to discuss some of Carl Jung's ideas about personality in the second half of life. His basic assumption is that middle age is the time during which we balance our personality—learn to do the things that come hardest for ourselves, learn to expand ourselves and become more complete. If introversion came the easiest, then in middle age social settings become easier. If one was naturally an extrovert, in middle age one better develops the reflective, solitary side of oneself. Having done either masculinity or femininity well, many individuals become more androgynous. How might Jung address the course of personality disorders in middle age?

2. *Class Activity.* Either write brief descriptions (such as a possible patient profile) for various personality disorders, or assign parts of this task to small groups. Then have teams guess the appropriate personality disorders for these descriptions. Assign points for correct guesses and award one team a "personality disorder detector award."

3. *Class Activity.* In small groups, have students analyze the most typical reinforcement schemes (types, sources, strategies) in their lives. What are some typical examples in their role as a college student? As a family member? What patterns are the most common in the small group? In the class?

4. *Class Demonstration.* Get a copy of the Narcissistic Personality Inventory by Robert Emmons that is given in this journal article: Emmons, R.A. 1987. Narcissism: Theory and measurement. *Journal of Personality and Social Psychology, 52,* 11-17. It measures narcissistic aspects in four areas: (1) leadership/authority; (2) self-absorption/self-admiration; (3) superiority/arrogance; and (4) exploitiveness/entitlement. Have students discuss these four aspects and discuss the amount of narcissism that is present in our culture today.

5. *Class Discussion.* Is narcissism becoming more common in America? Why? What role does narcissism play in the lives of politicians? Rock and movie stars? Business executives? Is there both a narcissistic style and a narcissistic personality disorder? What would the similarities and differences be?

6. *Class Activity.* Have small groups make a list of how they think Nancy the Narcissist and her twin sister Heloise the Histrionic would differ and how they would be the same, especially in how they might interact with people, behave during classtime, and determine and react to a crisis. Have groups share their lists.

7. *Class Discussion.* Do students find themselves in each of the personality disorders (problems with the medical student syndrome?)? If so, why does this happen? What criteria should be used to separate incidents of patterns with actually having the pattern? Passive-aggressive is a good choice to start discussion since everybody has acted out of this pattern but most are not in the whole personality disorder.

8. *Class Activity.* In small groups, do roleplays of an employee going to the human resources office or an employee assistance program for help in dealing with a boss who is (1) passive-aggressive; (2) narcissistic; (3) obsessive compulsive; (4) anti-social; and (5) histrionic. Although two people are assigned the helper and employee roles, others in the group can "feed appropriate lines." Do groups make good suggestions for dealing with an employer who has a personality disorder?

9. *Mini-Lecture.* **The Personality Disordered Workplace**
Sometimes unhealthy personalties are fostered by our work environments. For example, many workplaces help to create unhealthy workaholic patterns and many people end up entering counseling to be able to deal with the stresses caused by bosses whom workers label "tyrants, connivers, and bad-mouthers." In recent years, best-selling books have been written to deal with difficult bosses and companies (e.g., Schaef and Fassel's *The Addictive Organization* and Solomon's *Working with Difficult People*).

Schaef and Fassel suggest that workplaces can be addictive organizations and are characterized by features similar to those found in dysfunctional families that lead to addictions and personality disorders. These workplaces can be described as confusing, self-centered, dishonest, demanding perfectionism, denying, ethically deteriorated, spiritually bankrupt, chaotic, and crisis oriented. People working in imbalanced workplaces learn to cope by adapting unhealthy lifestyles such as workaholic, numbing and freezing all emotions, getting sick, drinking too much, and learning to deny reality.

In these workplaces, communication patterns are unreliable and rumors and gossip reign. Chaos is magnified by making many personnel changes as well as changes in the work processes themselves. Some administrators may allow themselves to be belligerent, vindictive, arrogant, deceitful, manipulative, and exploitative. Sexual harassment and other inappropriate behavioral patterns tend to be tolerated.

Schaef and Fassel believe that workplaces can be made healthy by adapting a twelve-step type program of change. It requires a long-term commitment to total change—and a move from control, dishonesty, and judgmentalism to one of flexibility, honesty, and mutual interactions.

When whole workplaces do not make a commitment to change, individuals can still change. Some choose to leave an unhealthy workplace and move on to a healthier one. Others change their strategies for working with the unhealthy components of the workplace. For example, Solomon defines many poor styles of bosses, colleagues, and subordinates and makes suggestions on how to better emotionally and behaviorally handle interactions with them. For example, Solomon suggests that bullies in the workplace are people who appear self-confident and strong but use belittlement and threats to keep control. She suggests standing up to them while being friendly and self-confident in order to avoid a clash of wills. Specifically, if one's boss is a bully, Solomon recommends (1) Letting the bully vent anger without attempting to stop the venting; (2) Dealing with the problem without criticizing the bullying; and (3) Don't gang up to make a complaint because this usually backfires. Her assumption is that bullies lose their power if you don't cower.

Of course, other individual solutions are possible too. An individual can reduce work stress by relaxation training, exercise, assessing and correcting irrational cognitions about work, and by self-limiting the number of hours that are spent on work.

10. *Class Discussion.* The book suggests that one current hypothesis draws parallels between post-traumatic stress disorder and the borderline personality disorder. What similarities and differences do you perceive in etiologies, symptoms, implications, and treatment?

11. *Class Activity.* The book describes three variants of paranoid personality: the paranoid-antisocial, the paranoid-narcissist, and the paranoid-compulsive. In small groups, have students develop three appropriate case studies for these variants. They should include (1) probable family backgrounds, (2) most striking symptoms and specific examples of how these symptoms are expressed, (3) typical effects of this maladaptive pattern on family, friends, and work, and (4) suggestions to the counselor.

12. *Class Discussion.* Schizotypal symptoms may include magical thinking, such as mind reading and clairvoyance, odd perceptions, such as hallucinations of talking with a dead friend, and other unusual thoughts. How are New Age/psychic persons and schizotypal persons alike? Different? Do you think that most psychic experiences are due to schizotypal personality disorder? If not, how could you detect the differences between someone with schizotypal personality disorder and a person with psychic abilities?

13. *Class Demonstration.* Share example items from Millon assessment scales for the personality disorders.

14. *Class Demonstration.* Have a speaker from Gamblers Anonymous or use some of their literature to address some of the issues involved in this impulsive disorder. The speaker may wish to address opinions about state government involvement in lottery games, casinos, and other forms of betting.

15. *Mini-Lecture.* **Cognitive Therapy and Personality Disorders**
Material for this mini-lecture comes from a 1990 book—*Cognitive Therapy of Personality Disorders* by Aaron Beck and Arthur Freeman (Chapter 3 is especially useful for expanding this mini-lecture). Students are familiar with the general assumptions of cognitive therapy because of its acceptance in the area of depression—that cognitions about loss add to depression. With personality disorders, too, individuals are susceptible to certain life experiences because of their cognitive errors and oversensitivity to one type of stress. For example, the narcissist focuses on trauma to one's self-esteem, and the dependent person is overly sensitive to loss of love and help.

Here, briefly, is a basic belief associated with each of the nine personality disorders as well as the major strategy in overt behavior. The dependent personality disorder believes "I am helpless" and so uses an attachment strategy. The avoidant personality disorder focuses on "I may get hurt" and uses an avoidance strategy. The passive-aggressive personality disorder utilizes a resistance strategy because of the core belief that "I could be stepped on." Paranoid personality disorder use a wariness strategy because "people are potential adversaries." The narcissistic personality disorder is associated with the attitude "I am special" and this attitude is accompanied by a self-aggrandizement strategy. The belief of the histrionic personality disorder is "I need to impress" and therefore the strategy is one of dramatics. Meanwhile, the obsessive compulsive personality disorder's basic belief is that "Errors are bad—I must not err" and adopts the perfectionism strategy. The antisocial personality disorder's basic belief is that "people are there to be taken" and the central strategy is attack. "I need plenty of space" is the schizoid's basic belief and therefore the strategy of isolation is used. Borderline personality disorder exhibits a wide range of typical beliefs and overt behavioral strategies and is better thought of in terms of ego deficit than in specific belief content. Schizotypal disorder is typified by peculiarities in thinking rather than an idiosyncratic basic belief.

Persons with personality disorders tend to have both overdeveloped and underdeveloped patterns due to their chosen strategy. For example, since obsessive compulsive personality disorder is the perfectionism strategy, the overdeveloped patterns are control, responsibility, and systematization while underdeveloped strategies are spontaneity and playfulness. The paranoid personality disorder leads to overdevelopment of vigilance, mistrust, and suspiciousness, and an underdevelopment of serenity, trust, and acceptance. Each personality disorder develops unique self-views and unique views about other people. For example, the obsessive compulsive personality disorder individual views the self as responsible for oneself and for others, has a fear of being overwhelmed, and demands perfectionism from the self to compensate for helplessness and defectiveness. Others are viewed as too casual, too self-indulgent, and too incompetent. The paranoid personality disordered person sees the self as righteous and mistreated by others and others as devious, deceptive, treacherous, and manipulative.

The cognitive therapist knows that the core beliefs of those with personality disorders are deeply ingrained and do not yield readily to cognitive techniques. Even when clients realize that their basic beliefs are dysfunctional, they are difficult to modify. Treatment takes a long time but there are spurts of improvement.

Chapter 18. Dissociative Disorders

Topic Overview:
I. Introduction

A. Memory
1. memory links past, present, and future, allowing recollections, organization, and future decisions
2. without a memory, one would always be starting over
3. memory provides identity, a sense of who one is

B. The Core of Dissociative Disorders
1. experiencing a breakdown in integration and self-recognition
2. significant alteration in memory or identity

II. Psychogenic Amnesia

A. Characteristics
1. suddenly unable to recall important personal information or past events in one's life
2. more extensive than normal forgetting
3. not attributable to an organic disorder and usually precipitated by extreme emotional stress

B. Kinds
1. localized or circumscribed amnesia is the most common type and involves forgetting all events over a limited time period
2. selective amnesia, the second most common form, is remembering only some events in a time period
3. amnestic episode is the forgotten or partially forgotten period and individuals often act puzzled, confused, and aimless
4. generalized amnesia is not remembering events and people in one's life yet retaining skills such as driving a car
5. continuous amnesia, which is rare, involves being unable to retain new experiences as they occur

C. Conditions of Occurrence
1. during wartime or in natural disasters
2. when one's health or safety is significantly threatened
3. 5-15% of mental disorders during combat are psychogenic amnesia
4. also after sudden losses or with guilt about immoral or sinful behavior

D. Personal Impact
    1. depends on the extent and importance of what is forgotten
    2. more difficulties when major life changes going on

III. Psychogenic Fugue

  A. Characteristics
    1. loss of memory and actual physical flight
    2. forget their personal identity and all details of past life
    3. travel a short distance, few social contacts, incomplete new identity
    4. may last only hours or days and end suddenly
    5. occasionally quite extensive and a well-integrated new identity, which is often more outgoing and less inhibited

  B. Conditions of Occurrence
    1. usually follows a severely stressful event or personal stress
    2. common characteristics of precipitating events: (1) inescapable perceived danger; (2) perceived loss of important objects; (3) overwhelming homicidal or suicidal impulses
    3. some adolescent runaways
    4. end abruptly with person awakening in an unfamiliar place or discovered by others

  C. Personal Impact
    1. most regain all their memories and have no more occurrences
    2. many forget events of the fugue period
    3. mostly brief and totally reversible
    4. longer fugues have more adjustment concerns
    5. some people commit illegal or violent acts in their fugue state and must face consequences

IV. Multiple Personality Disorder

  A. Introduction
    1. two or more distinct personalities, often called subpersonalities, with unique memories, behaviors, thoughts, and emotions
    2. the primary, or host, personality, appears more often than the others
    3. transition from one subpersonality to another is usually sudden and often dramatic
    4. transitions usually precipitated by stressful events
    5. first reported four centuries ago
    6. rare, but more common than once believed
    7. usually develops in early childhood but not diagnosed until adolescence or later
    8. 97% have been physically, often sexually, abused during their early years
    9. 4 to 9 times more common in women

B. The Subpersonalities
   1. mutually amnesic relationships are when subpersonalities have no awareness of the others
   2. mutually cognizant patterns are when each subpersonality is well aware of others and may even talk among themselves
   3. most common is one-way amnesic relationship when some subpersonalities are aware of others but awareness is not reciprocated
   4. co-conscious subpersonalities are those that have awareness and they watch the actions and thoughts of other subpersonalities but do not interact with them
   5. at first thought most were two or three subpersonalities but average now considered to be 13 or 14, often emerging in groups of 2 or 3 at a time
   6. subpersonalities usually have their own names
   7. they differ in personality styles
   8. differ in age, sex, race, and family history
   9. different abilities, including different handwriting styles, tastes in food, friends, music, and literature preferences
   10. differ in physiological responses, such as autonomic nervous system activity, blood pressure levels, and menstrual cycles

C. The Prevalence of Multiple Personality Disorder
   1. by 1970 only 100 cases ever reported, but increasing rapidly now
   2. growing belief in the authenticity of the disorder
   3. a common symptom is losses of time throughout one's life
   4. some multiple personality cases were incorrectly diagnosed as schizophrenia
   5. still average four diagnoses before multiple personality disorder

V. Explanations of Dissociative Disorders

A. The Psychodynamic View
   1. extreme use of repression
   2. parents overreact to child's expressions of id impulses, children become excessively afraid of these impulses, and when they violate their moral code may be unable to face this unacceptable situation
   3. come to fear the world as dangerous and take flight symbolically by pretending to be another person looking on from afar

B. The Behavioral View
   1. acquired through operant conditioning
   2. a way to avoid extreme anxiety
   3. a subtle reinforcement process rather than a hard-working unconscious

C. State-Dependent Learning
   1. remember best when returned to the same state or situation of learning
   2. psychological states as well as physiological ones
   3. arousal levels are an important part of memory processes
   4. in multiple personality disorders, different arousal levels may elicit different clusters of memories, thoughts, and abilities

D. Self-hypnosis
  1. hypnotic amnesia
  2. dissociative disorders as a form of self-hypnosis
  3. consciously or unconsciously hypnotize the self into forgetting horrifying experiences
  4. multiple personality disorders begin at 4 to 6 in highly suggestible children
  5. various explanations can be offered for how self-hypnosis might occur, from it being a special trance, utilizing attention and expectation, or diverting and then refocusing attention

VI. Treatments for Psychogenic Amnesia and Fugue

  A. Psychodynamic Therapy
    1. free associate to try to make forgotten experiences conscious
    2. may be the most appropriate and effective approach

  B. Hypnotic Therapy
    1. in conjunction with or instead of psychodynamic therapy
    2. use hypnosis to guide recall of forgotten events

  C. Intravenous Injections
    1. sodium amobarbital or sodium pentobarbitaol
    2. lowers inhibitions
    3. brief use or physical dependence occurs

VII. Treatments for Multiple Personality Disorder

  A. Rarely Spontaneous Recovery

  B. Therapeutic Process
    1. recovering memory gaps
    2. recognizing full breadth of the disorder
    3. integrating the subpersonalities

  C. Getting Subpersonalities to Want Integration

  D. Full Integration May Not Be Needed

VIII. Depersonalization Disorder

  A. Symptoms
    1. alteration in one's experience of the self in which one's mental functioning or body feels unreal or foreign
    2. doubling, or sensation of floating a few feet above
    3. body distortions
    4. "dreamlike" emotional state
    5. sense of unreality in sensory experiences, mental operations, and behavior
    6. derealization, or feeling the external world is unreal and strange

B. Other Criteria
   1. transient depersonalization experiences are common but depersonalization disorder is not
   2. occurs mostly from young children through young adulthood
   3. can also occur after meditation or when traveling to new places
   4. depersonalization disorder is persistent, recurrent, causes marked distress and impairment
   5. precipitated by extreme fatigue, physical pain, intense stress, anxiety, depression, or recovery from substance abuse
   6. not only chronic, but improvement may be only temporary with symptoms returning under mild anxiety

C. Explanations
   1. few theoretical explanations
   2. psychodynamic theorists suggest primitive, highly pathological defense mechanism
   3. cognitive theorists suggest imbalance of focus between internal and external events
   4. more prone if excessively attentive to bodily sensations and inner thoughts

IX. Dissociative Disorders: The State of the Field

A. Growing Numbers

B. Increase in Research

C. Lots of Media Interest

D. Some Inaccurate Diagnosing Due to Popularity

Learning Objectives:
1. Know what aspects are shared by all dissociative disorders.
2. Define psychogenic amnesia and be able to distinguish among the four kinds: localized, selective, generalized, and continuous.
3. Describe the typical pattern of psychogenic fugue.
4. Describe the features of multiple personality disorder and be able to define primary personality and the three types of subpersonalities: mutually amnesic, mutually cognizant, and one-way amnesic.
5. Define iatrogenic.
6. Describe the psychodynamic explanation of dissociative disorders.
7. Describe the behavioral explanation of dissociative disorders.
8. Explain the possible role of state-dependent learning in dissociative disorders.
9. Explain the possible role of self-hypnosis in dissociative disorders and summarize research studies in this area.
10. Describe the possible roles of hypnosis and trauma in the development of multiple personalities.
11. Describe typical treatment techniques for persons with dissociative disorders, including free association, hypnosis, and sodium amobarbital.
12. Compare and contrast depersonalization and derealization.
13. Distinguish depersonalization disorder from the other dissociative disorders.

Instruction Suggestions:

1. *Class Discussion.* If you have any current or former soap opera buffs in your class, you may be able to get examples of dissociative disorders from favored soap opera plots (if a current storyline includes amnesia, fugue, or multiple personality, you might want to videotape a few pertinent scenes and show them to the class). *The Bold and the Beautiful* had Stephanie lose her memory and go from riches to rags and spend time as a homeless individual. Several years ago Dr. David Stewart on *As the World Turns* experienced a fugue state and went from being a medical researcher to a pharmacist. The now-defunct *The Doctors* had Dr. Althea Davis experience psychogenic amnesia in three different storylines over the years. What examples can they give? Any examples from prime-time television? You can even add to your lectures, "Psychogenic fugues are rare, that is, except in daytime TV." If students (or you) can come up with detailed examples, discuss whether the disorders are accurately shown.

2. *Class Demonstration.* Videotape and show to your class a few brief scenes from movies that deal with multiple personality disorder. For example, you can use *Three Faces of Eve* and *Sybil.* You can even contrast a specific movie scene with how it is done in the book. Discuss the scenes and passages.

3. *Class Discussion.* Discuss why multiple personality diagnosis has gone from "doesn't exist" to increased diagnosis. What reasons do students think provide the best explanation?

4. *Class Demonstration.* Compare some passages from *Three Faces of Eve* with *I'm Eve.*

5. *Class Demonstration.* Talk shows and TV newsmagazines often cover dramatic cases of amnesia, fugue, and multiple personality. It might be worth it to tape and show a portion of one of these programs.

6. *Class Discussion.* A man has been convicted of rape due to knowingly seducing a multiple personality's subpersonality incapable of being able to consent to sexual intercourse. What do you think of this decision? If you were on the jury, what criteria would you have used?

7. *Class Discussion.* Schizophrenia is no longer the "wastebasket" diagnostic category. With increases in diagnosing multiple personality disorder, post-traumatic stress disorder, and borderline personality disorder, are any of these the "new wastebasket"? One professional says, "Beware of any diagnosis becoming popular enough to be known by an acronym," i.e., MPD, PTSD, and BPD.

Topic Overview:
I. Early and Middle Adulthood

    A. Daniel Levinson's Theory
        1. early adulthood, from 22 to 40 years, characterized by high energy, contradiction, stress, establishing a niche, choosing aspirations
        2. middle adulthood, from 45 to 60 years, characterized as personally satisfying and socially valuable yet with growing biological problems, numerous responsibilities, and dealing with upcoming old age
        3. most stress in the transitions between the major stages
        4. early adult transition, from 17 to 22 years, is an unsettled time with modified family relations and insecure efforts
        5. middle life transition, from 40 to 45 years, is a period of significant changes in which persons no longer feel young and vibrant yet also become more passionate, reflective, and accepting
        6. middle life transition may be referred to as midlife crisis
        7. 80% of men in Levinson's interviews reported middle life transition as tumultuous and painful and involving anxiety and depression

    B. Effects of Cohorts
        1. cohorts are people born in the same era or generation
        2. affected by the historical and personal events to which one is exposed
        3. cohort groups establish relevant values, expectations, and timetables
        4. persons "in sync" with their cohorts experience less stress and tension

II. Old Age

    A. Defining Old Age
        1. arbitrarily defined as 65 years or older, which is 13% of the United States population
        2. young-old from 65 to 74, old-old from 75 to 84, and oldest-old from 85 and up
        3. life expectancy in the United States has increased in the 20th century due to better health care and better life habits

    B. Circumstances
        1. older men are nearly twice as likely to be married as older women, with half of all older women being widows
        2. two-thirds live with at least one family member and nearly one-third live alone
        3. majority own their own home and only 5% are in nursing homes

4. 90% are Caucasian, 8% African-American
5. about half live in nine states
6. have more health problems than younger people, with 29% saying they have poor health

C. Defining Age Concepts
1. chronological age is number of years one has lived since birth
2. functional age is based on biological, social, and psychological age
3. biological age is one's present position with respect to one's potential life span and is assessed by functioning of vital organ systems
4. social age is based on one's roles, habits, and behaviors
5. psychological age refers to one's capacity to adapt behavior to a changing environment
6. many older people are stereotyped

III. Successful Aging: A Stress-and-Coping Model

A. Change and Stress
1. wear and tear leading to being prone to illness
2. taking control over key risk factors so that prudent living and good use of health technology leads to better long lives

B. Richard Lazarus' Stress-and-Coping Model
1. primary appraisal to judge stressfulness of a situation
2. secondary appraisal to judge what might and can be done in response
3. reappraisals in which one adjusts perceptions and behaviors
4. older people use a wide range of strategies to cope with negative life events and these can be described as either problem-focused or emotion-focused
5. another strategy is a spiritual strategy

C. Alleviating Stress
1. respond well to cognitive and behavioral therapies for depression, anxiety disorders, atypical bereavement, and chronic functional limitations
2. cognitive and behavioral therapies are generally accepted and less threatening than traditional therapies and do not have health risks of psychotropic medications

IV. Common Clinical Syndromes in the Aging

A. Statistics
1. 50% of elderly could benefit from mental health services yet fewer than 20% receive help
2. some elderly have a highly stigmatized view of mental health problems
3. limited insurance reimbursements to providers of mental health care

B. Depression
1. most common mental health problem of older adults
2. between 1 and 20% of older adults meet DSM-III-R criteria for clinical depression

3. best assessed in a structured clinical interview than in a self-report questionnaire, although Geriatric Depression Scale and Beck Depression Inventory may be helpful
4. need to look for organic causes so use neurological assessment or Folstein's Mini-Mental State Examination
5. antidepressants often used but drug processing is different in older people
6. use of cognitive-behavior therapy or brief psychodynamic therapy
7. family therapy is useful because many families unintentionally reinforce negative adaptive behaviors
8. electroconvulsive therapy (ECT) has been used often with the elderly
9. depression often accompanied by suicidal thoughts or actions
10. use of psychoeducational programs for elderly and for their care-giving family members

C. Anxiety Disorders
   1. anxiety often coexists with depression and may be hard to determine which is the major disorder
   2. generalized anxiety disorder about 7%, agoraphobia from 2 to 5%, simple phobias from 1 to 12%, and panic disorders in less than 1%
   3. use of antianxiety medication needing lower doses and with higher risk for side effects
   4. can use relaxation training, systematic desensitization, and anxiety management techniques

D. Cognitive Impairments
   1. dementia is an organic mental syndrome with impaired cognitive functioning in areas such as memory, abstract thinking, and judgment
   2. evidence of unusually severe impairment in short- and long-term memory
   3. one or more of the following: impaired abstract thinking, impaired judgment, impaired performance on simple psychomotor tests, noticeable personality changes
   4. disturbances significantly interfere with occupational or typical social activities
   5. evidence from medical history, physical exam, or lab tests that there is an organic basis
   6. at 65, 2-4%; over 80, about 30%
   7. metabolic or nutritional disorders, sensory dysfunctions
   8. Alzheimer's disease is most common dementia and is a gradually progressive degenerative process that takes a 2- to 15-year course
   9. Alzheimer's begins with mild memory problems and attention lapses and leads to difficulty in completing complicated tasks and then difficulty with simple tasks and personality changes
   10. added anxiety and depression about the impaired thinking but later less concern about losses and then increased disorientation, wandering, poor judgment, and sleeping
   11. multi-infarct dementia is second most common and is due to strokes
   12. Pick's disease and Jakob-Creutzfeldt disease are rare progressive dementias
   13. Huntington's chorea has its onset during middle adulthood and is caused by dominant gene inheritance
   14. both acetylcholine and L-glutamate are depleted in Alzheimer's
   15. possibly a genetic basis
   16. viral agent could be involved, as it is in Jakob-Creutzfeldt dementia

17. possible role of toxic substances
18. use of behavioral interventions, including addition of more pleasant activities
19. stress of caregiving—financial and emotional and need for support groups
20. concern with abuses in the nursing-home industry

E. Substance Abuse
   1. hard to determine prevalence in the elderly
   2. about 5% of older males have alcohol-related problem
   3. there are both early-onset drinkers who are now old and late-onset alcohol abusers, whose drinking problems start in their fifties or later
   4. the intentional or inadvertent misuse of prescription drugs
   5. among persons who receive prescriptions from a physician, the average number of prescriptions is 7.5, but it is 14.2 for those over 60
   6. special AA groups called Golden Years

F. Delirium and Psychotic Disorders
   1. most older schizophrenics require some structured care
   2. the rare delusional disorder is slightly more common with age

V. Other Factors in the Mental Health of the Elderly

A. Ethnicity
   1. ethnic group is a collection of people who share some common ancestry, memories of specific, unique historical events, and a cultural focus
   2. "double jeopardy" is being old and a member of a minority racial or ethnic group; "triple jeopardy" is old, minority, and female
   3. language barrier and cultural beliefs may prevent seeking mental health and medical services

B. Long-Term Care
   1. majority have at least one chronic health problem
   2. 5% in nursing homes, but many others fear being put in one
   3. health insurance plans do not cover costs of permanent placement

C. Health Maintenance
   1. following health habits and managing stress
   2. better health and also a buffer against depression

VI. Problems of Aging: The State of the Field

A. New Focus of Attention

B. Identification of Special Concerns of the Aged

C. Dealing with Caretaking Pressures

D. Emphasis on Prevention and Preparation

Learning Objectives:
1. Describe the domain and goals of geropsychology.
2. Explain the role of psychological stress in the lives of older people and describe Lazarus and Folkman's stress-and-coping model.
3. Know which counseling techniques have been shown to be most helpful with older patients.
4. Describe the attitudes of elderly persons toward mental health problems and of clinicians toward treating the elderly.
5. Describe the prevalence of depression among older adults and evaluate the effectiveness of various treatments.
6. Describe the prevalence, diagnosis, and treatment of anxiety disorders among elderly people.
7. Define dementia and list six different kinds of dementia among the elderly.
8. Compare and contrast neurotransmitter, genetic, and infectious agent explanations of Alzheimer's disease.
9. Describe and evaluate interventions done with Alzheimer's patients and their family members.
10. Discuss alcohol abuse and prescription drug abuse and treatment among older persons.
11. Know the prevalence of schizophrenia and paranoid disorders among the elderly.
12. Discuss societal factors that contribute to mental disorders among the elderly, including discrimination, quality of long-term care facilities, and inadequate health maintenance.

Instruction Suggestions:
1. *Class Demonstration.* Students can better absorb the ideas of Erikson (presented in Chapter 19) and Levinson about adulthood development if you visually chart out (on the blackboard, with a transparency, in a handout) the two theories together to make easier comparisons of timing and critical tasks. Have students discuss the similarities and differences in these two major theories.

2. *Class Discussion.* Describe the empty-nest syndrome of middle age. Discuss how it used to be considered a source of depression and now is associated with an emotional uplift. Have students discuss why attitudes toward the empty-nest syndrome have changed since the 1950s. What does this mean about attitudes toward family? Aging? Also, it used to be considered a female phenomenon and now is descriptive of both men and women. Why?

3. *Lecture Additions.* Through the DSM-II classification systems, one of the possible diagnoses was *involutional melancholia,* a type of depression that did not occur until middle age and was primarily seen in females. Various explanations were offered for this overwhelming and severe depression. Some psychologists and physicians thought it was caused by hormonal changes associated with menopause. If males did experience involutional melancholia, it appeared later (in one's sixties instead of one's fifties) and did not appear as dramatically because hormonal changes due to aging were more gradual for males. Other explanations centered around the empty-nest syndrome. Once women lost their value as mothers, their lives were empty and without much meaning and severe depression resulted. Changes in society and the field of psychiatry led to the dismissal of involutional melancholia in the DSM-III.

4. *Mini-Lecture.* **Psychological Masquerading**

You have already learned about psychological disorders that mask as medical problems—conversion disorders, somatization, and somatoform pain are examples. Yet, there are also cases when organically caused disorders are misdiagnosed as psychological problems because professionals miss signs of organic syndrome. Psychological masquerading refers to this situation.

Symptoms of depression, agitation, memory impairment, hallucinations, and poor judgment can indeed be indicators of mental disorders, but they may also be indicators of some medical problem. One graduate student, for example, had all the symptoms of an anxiety disorder—sleep disorder, change in appetite, sweating, pounding heart, weight loss, and so forth. Her friends thought that she had plenty of things that contributed to her anxiety. She was both working on a massive research project and writing a major paper. In addition, as a foreign student, all of her family support system was a couple of thousand miles away. However, a medical doctor was able to pick out a couple of features that did not match a typical anxiety reaction. First, her eyes now seemed to bulge right out of her head (like a goldfish's eyes), her hair had become thinner and more brittle, and her appetite was huge yet she was losing weight regularly. Finally, instead of the cold sweat typical of anxiety, she broke out in a warm sweat. This student's problem was hyperthyroidism rather than an anxiety disorder.

Another example of psychological masquerading is the story of the composer George Gershwin. At the height of his career, Gershwin began to experience headaches, irritability, memory problems, and many symptoms that are typical of being stressed. His brother and friends indeed thought that Gershwin was overwhelmed with adjusting to fame, overwork, and a new personal relationship. Indeed, they referred to him as a hypochondriac or as a person demanding attention. His symptoms became worse and included sensitivity to light, numbness, and unrelenting headaches. He sometimes fell, and an acquaintance who was with him once when he fell remarked, "Oh, just let him lie there—he just wants the attention." Finally he was taken seriously and hospitalized. Within a few days he fell into a coma and an operation revealed a malignant brain tumor. He died the next day.

Sometimes drug-induced problems are missed and diagnosed as schizophrenia or dementia. A young male was diagnosed as schizophrenic, but an alert counselor noticed that the man had mainly visual hallucinations. Visual hallucinations are more common with organic disorders and auditory hallucinations are more common with schizophrenia (though they are not exclusive); the counselor asked the man more questions and discovered the chronic abuse of amphetamines had caused the symptoms. A concerned daughter of a woman recovering from health problems in a nursing home found that her aged mother's apparent dementia was really due to interactions from 28 prescription medications that her mother was taking. When a professional readjusted her mother's medications, the disorientation, memory impairment, and poor judgment were alleviated.

Obviously, few counselors are experts in diagnosing medical problems. They do need to learn to observe symptoms that make them suspicious of psychological masquerading. They can do some simple neurological assessment and make appropriate referrals when physical problems are a possibility. Often, individuals with organic disorders have trouble drawing simple three-dimensional figures, drawing the face of a clock, remembering three simple objects for even five minutes, and doing simple calculations (e.g., what is left when 7 is subtracted from 22? What is one-third of twelve?).

5. *Class Project.* Have students interview an older person, asking them about their dreams, life views, fears, biggest accomplishments, worst problems faced, typical coping strategies, and so forth. You might have your students come up with the list of questions to ask all persons. You might want to pre-arrange permission for students to interview individuals in a nearby nursing home, congregate meal site, or community senior citizen's center. Either have students discuss the interviews or turn in a written report.

6. *Lecture Additions.* You might mention how older adults alleviate stress and depression by having contact with pets or children and by volunteering in their community.

7. *Class Demonstration.* Bring to class copies of Geriatric Depression Scale, Beck Depression Inventory, and/or Folstein's Mini-Mental State Examination. Share some of the items and discuss why the author has suggested that these measures are appropriate for use with an elderly population.

8. *Class Discussion.* Propose that there is a Caregiver Syndrome Disorder that is experienced by middle-aged adults who are taking care of both their own children and their aging parents. Have the class discuss what the main symptoms of CSD would be, and have them develop an appropriate treatment package.

9. *Class Discussion.* Discuss the reasons why the elderly receive more medications and ECT than psychotherapy. Is it due to professional bias? Beliefs of the elderly clients? What is your opinion of appropriate treatments for the aged?

10. *Class Discussion.* Have the class discuss whether Alzheimer's disease research should be a higher priority for government funding. How about other diseases among the aged? Should we put more money into Alzheimer's research or into AIDS research (assuming only one can be increased)?

11. *Lecture Additions.* Under Huntington's chorea, you can mention that the folksinger Woody Guthrie died of Huntington's chorea. You can also discuss the availability of genetic testing for this disease yet most family members choose not to take the test.

12. *Class Discussion.* One very noted case was a doctor who used a suicide machine to aid a woman with Alzheimer's disease to commit suicide. How do students feel about individuals with Alzheimer's killing themselves during the early stages of the disease before they lose most of their abilities?

13. *Class Activity.* Draw a long line on the blackboard. At the left end mark "conception," and at the other end mark "age at death." Have students copy this line in their notebooks. Tell them to mark an X where they currently are on this line. Have them also jot down a number answer for "How old do you think you will be when you die?" and also "How old would you like to be when you die?" Discuss these answers, perhaps in small groups.

14. *Class Demonstration.* Have a health care administrator of a nursing home speak to your class about the needs of their elderly population. As an alternative, you can visit a nursing home or retirement community.

15. *Class Discussion.* Have students discuss what it means to be an "adult-child" vs. an "adult-orphan."

Topic Overview:
I. Clinical Influences on the Criminal Justice System

    A. Basic Definitions
       1. criminal commitment for being judged mentally unstable at the time of the crime
       2. criminal commitment for being judged mentally unstable at the time of the trial

    B. Criminal Commitment and Insanity during Commission of a Crime
       1. John Hinckley example
       2. M'Naghten rule established in 1843 of not knowing nature and quality of the behavior or not knowing what one is doing is wrong
       3. alternative is irresistible impulse test first used in 1834
       4. Durham test established by Supreme Court in 1954 of not being responsible if the crime was a product of mental disease or mental defect
       5. 1955 American Law Institute guidelines using elements of all three tests
       6. after Hinckley verdict guidelines made stricter
       7. revised criminal insanity test in 1983 also used in half of the states
       8. three states have no insanity plea
       9. majority acquitted by insanity are diagnosed as schizophrenic and hospitalized
      10. successful insanity pleas more often by whites and females
      11. critics as to compatibility of law and behavioral science, workability of mental health standards, and possibly letting dangerous criminals escape
      12. only 1 in 1,000 cases involves an insanity plea
      13. often successful insanity plea leads to more confinement in hospital than would have been confined in a prison
      14. trend toward "guilty but mentally ill"
      15. some states use "guilty with diminished responsibility"
      16. some states use a sex-offender status

    C. Criminal Commitment and Incompetence to Stand Trial
       1. inability to aid in preparation and conduct of one's defense due to mental disorder
       2. on side of caution so that convictions can not be appealed on this ground
       3. has sometimes been abused and confined individuals for long periods without a trial
       4. Jackson v. Indiana in 1972 ruled chronically disordered defendants cannot be indefinitely committed under criminal status
       5. used to mean use of maximum security institutions for the criminally insane but now includes even outpatient treatment

II. Legal Influences on the Mental Health System

   A. Civil Commitment
      1. many involuntarily committed each year
      2. some states give greater protection to suspected criminals than to suspected psychotics
      3. general guidelines of need of treatment and dangerous to oneself or others
      4. use parens patriae for state to make involuntary hospitalization to promote the individual's best interests and protect from self-harm or self-neglect
      5. use police power to protect society from harm from a violent person
      6. statutes vary from state to state
      7. most formal commitment proceedings initiated by family members and procedure is simple if a minor involved
      8. in 1979, Addington v. Texas outlined the minimum standard of proof necessary for commitment
      9. can do emergency commitment with many state laws using two-physician certificates
     10. professionals poor at predicting violence and suicide
     11. most likely to be violent is person hallucinating and exhibiting little emotional withdrawal
     12. criticisms include problems defining mental illness and dangerousness, misuse of civil commitment, and that involuntary treatment does not produce the best results
     12. acceptance of broad involuntary commitment statutes peaked in 1962 when Supreme Court encouraged mental health facilities instead of prisons for those with unacceptable behavior
     13. use of imminent dangerousness, which encourages use of short-term predictions of dangerousness

   B. Protecting Patients' Rights
      1. without treatment, mental institutions are merely prisons for the unconvicted
      2. in 1972, Wyatt v. Stickney established institutions' obligation to provide adequate   treatment to all involuntarily committed
      3. in 1975, O'Connor v. Donaldson established that those who can safely survive in freedom cannot be confined
      4. in 1982, Youngberg v. Romeo supported the right to treatment
      5. Protection and Advocacy for Mentally Ill Individuals Act in 1986
      6. dealing with right to treatment, right to freedom, and homelessness
      7. most right-to-refuse-treatment rulings have centered on biological treatments
      8. some states acknowledge patient's right to refuse electroconvulsive therapy, or at least to get additional consent
      9. with more being known about side effects of psychotropic medications, more are seeing a need to allow patients the right to refuse these medicines
     10. in 1973, Sounder v. Brennan said that working patients should be paid
     11. other cases deal with the right to be in less restrictive facilities
     12. rulings can disrupt effectiveness of behavioral token economy programs

III. Other Clinical-Legal Interactions

  A. Malpractice Suits
     1. 16% of psychiatrists, and fewer other counselors, have been sued
     2. cases of improper termination of treatment
     3. civil malpractice suits capable of having significant effects on clinical decisions

  B. Jury Selection
     1. jury specialists who make recommendations for how to pick jury members
     2. validity undetermined

  C. The Scope of Clinical Practice
     1. less clear boundaries among the helping professions
     2. 1989 Congress passed bills that permitted psychologists to treat elderly and
        disabled people
     3. DOD exploring training to allow Army psychologists to prescribe drugs
     4. role of lobbying

IV. Self-Regulation: Ethics and the Mental Health Field

  A. Clinician Obstacles
     1. complex questions without obvious answers
     2. clinicians may not appreciate or may ignore the system in which they work
     3. some clinicians are self-serving or immoral
     4. having and updating ethical guidelines

  B. APA Ethics Code
     1. revised in 1981 and amended in 1990
     2. dealing with the media issues, such as self-help books and radio shows
     3. research ethics
     4. not exploiting clients and students

  C. Sexual Misconduct
     1. surveys of therapists having sexual relationships with clients
     2. either decreasing over the last decade or less open on surveys
     3. neither sexual relations with clients or former clients, although some would put a
        time restriction on the latter situation
     4. sexual fantasies of patients on occasion

  D. Confidentiality
     1. a very important feature of therapy
     2. discussion with supervisor
     3. outpatients who are clearly dangerous, even homicidal
     4. legitimate and ethical to break confidentiality to prevent danger

V. Mental Health, Business, and Economics

  A. Business and Mental Health
     1. more closely working together
     2. employee assistance programs
     3. stress-reduction and problem-solving seminars

151

B. Economics and Mental Health
   1. wanting to reduce expenses influenced deinstitutionalization programs
   2. increased funding for mental health services from $3.3 billion in 1969 to $18.5 billion in 1989, but not an increase per person seeking therapy
   3. many more now seek services
   4. peer review system

VI. The Person within the Profession

A. Therapist
   1. own needs and preferences and theoretical orientations
   2. personal leanings sometimes overcome professional standards
   3. many go into therapy as clients
   4. imposter phenomenon felt by majority at times

B. Goals: Understand, Predict, and Alter Abnormal Functioning

VII. Law, Society, and the Mental Health Profession: The State of the Field

A. Activities Tied to Other Societal Institutions

B. Remarkable Increase in Societal Acceptance

C. Healthy System of Checks and Balances

D. Dealing with Profession's Strengths and Weaknesses

Learning Objectives:
1. Summarize the interaction between the mental health profession and government.
2. Know what is involved in criminal commitment and distinguish among guidelines based on the M'Naghten rule, irresistible impulse, and the Durham test.
3. Evaluate the effectiveness of the insanity defense.
4. Explain mental incompetence to stand trial and typical consequences.
5. Explain the process of civil commitment and provide the criteria for involuntary commitment as defined by Addington v. Texas.
6. Discuss patient right to treatment, right to refuse treatment, and other established patient rights.
7. Discuss the issue of malpractice suits against therapists.
8. Explain how lawyers use mental health professionals.
9. Explain how legislative and judicial systems affect the scope of clinical practice.
10. Discuss the code of ethics for psychologists.
11. Explain how Tarasoff v. Regents of the University of California clarified when therapists should break confidentiality.
12. Discuss the relationship between clinical practice and the business world.

Instruction Suggestions:

1. *Class Activity.* Develop some court case scenarios in which mental disorders play a role in the trial. You can create your own or, over time, develop synopses based on real cases. Have small groups wrestle with the issue of whether juries should use the information about the mental illness and how they think it should affect the trial outcome. You might see if there is consensus across groups, what kinds of cases lead to successful insanity pleas, and so forth. A few possibilities include a man who knowingly sexually abuses a childlike subpersonality of a multiple personality disorder patient, a case of assault on a hot summer day at the beach in which the defendant claims PTSD from Desert Storm was the cause, a serial murder who hacks apart his victims and cannibalizes them, a kidnap victim who is confined and subjected to "brainwashing" techniques for fifty days, then commits a crime with the group holding her hostage, a battered spouse who ends up killing the batterer and claims she feared for her life, and a teenager who says his crime is due to the mental disorder of cocaine abuse and requests treatment instead of juvenile detention center.

2. *Class Discussion.* Have the class generate a list of criteria that might be used to determine if one is insane—then turn the task around and have them generate a list of criteria that could be used to determine that one is sane. Which is the more difficult list to establish?

3. *Class Discussion.* Have your students discuss the advantages and disadvantages of each of the three rules determining acquittal of a criminal defendant by reason of insanity. Which of the three is best? What features would they use to develop the best model of all?

4. *Class Discussion.* Have the class debate the advisability of using "guilty but mentally ill" or "guilty with diminished responsibility" for individuals accused of drug crimes (possession, intent to sell, public intoxication). What would be the implication for sentencing?

5. *Class Discussion.* Generate a list of characteristics that might indicate incompetence to stand trial. How does this list compare to one that would determine insanity? What are the primary circumstances under which persons should be committed?

6. *Class Demonstration.* Have a legal or mental health professional who has been involved in making civil commitments address your class. In addition to talking about the actual procedures and providing examples of when commitment is appropriate, ask the speaker to address how they deal with the emotional aspects of making involuntary commitments.

7. *Class Discussion.* Addington v. Texas (1979) established that there were minimum standards of proof necessary for commitment. What are your students' ideas about what is "clear and convincing" proof?

8. *Lecture Additions.* In 1991, both the National Alliance for the Mentally Ill and the American Psychological Association published articles that stated that many mentally ill patients are being held indefinitely in jails rather than being committed to mental health facilities. In some cases, mentally ill individuals have been "lost" in the correctional system for months without a hearing, trial, or treatment.

9. *Lecture Additions.* When lecturing about the current grounds for involuntary commitment, you might wish to address examples of abuse before modern standards were established. There are cases from the 1950s of parents committing pregnant teenage daughters to mental hospitals because "our daughter is a good girl so she must be mentally ill to have gotten herself pregnant," the infant being adopted out of the hospital, and professionals neglecting to release the female for sometimes as long as several years.

10. *Lecture Additions.* There have been incidences that when mental health advocates have questioned the high dosage of medicines for a patient the patient has been switched to medications that are stronger—because then the numbers go down and the appearance is that the patient is getting less medicine. One could be switched, for example, from Thorazine to Haldol.

11. *Class Demonstration.* Read a variety of examples from the *APA Ethics Casebook* and have the class guess the rulings in these cases.

12. *Class Discussion.* What consequences should there be for therapists who have sex with their clients (therapist = the rapist)? Should they lose their license? Should they be prosecuted for sexual abuse or rape? When would it be okay for a therapist to develop a relationship with a former client?

13. *Class Demonstration.* Have a speaker come from an Employee Assistance Program and tell about working in this setting.

Especially for New Teachers

Read over the following suggestions; you might use some of them to aid you in developing, organizing, and teaching your abnormal psychology course.

1. Before you do anything else, think about your personal teaching philosophy and views on psychology. How much of yourself do you wish to incorporate into the structure of the course? How are your going to translate your own values and goals into teaching, grading, and interacting with students? Are there beliefs that you want to emphasize and others that you want to minimize?

2. Prepare your course well in advance of the course starting date if at all possible. Two of the first things to get done are (1) ordering desirable media and (2) constructing a course syllabus.

3. Students like it if you can provide them with copies of the syllabus on the first day of class. It is wise to run off several extra copies so that you can provide students with a second copy if they lose their original, have copies for students that late-add your class, and have an extra copy for an interested colleague.

4. Make your syllabus as detailed and as informative as possible. It is like giving students a road map of the course—if you tell them where you are headed and the landmarks along the way they are much more likely to reach the final destination with you. Things that you might include in the course syllabus include: textbook assignments (including dates), test dates and which chapters are on each test (if you cannot be sure of the exact date of a test remember that it is better to give a test later than the originally scheduled date than before), make-up test procedures and consequences of missing project due dates, written assignments (what they are, how to do them, when they are due, how much they count), grading scale, course objectives, class attendance policy, extra credit possibilities, a statement about plagiarism (define it) and cheating, office hours, test styles (e.g., multiple choice, essay). Read over your first draft as if you were a student in the class and adjust what you have written to be more complete and in an appropriate tone.

5. Decide whether you want to lecture each class period or utilize discussion, exercises, media, and other special activities in addition to your lectures. If you want to use guest speakers, arrange for them well in advance.

6. What test format do you wish to use? Decide on the basis of goals (e.g., essay questions require more thought processing; multiple-choice and true-false questions can allow immediate feedback), and practicalities (e.g., multiple-choice questions can be quickly scored even with large classes).

7. Do you wish to try anything different with your testing and evaluation? You might try letting students have copies of an entire test bank (without answers); they learn a lot trying to figure out the answers to the entire potential item pool. Or, with classes of thirty, you might grade their multiple-choice tests as they finish, allow them to review their errors, and therefore be better prepared for a make-up/retake exam offered during the final exam period.

8. Decide whether you want to inform students about what is likely to be on a test. You may wish to say nothing so that students must either learn everything or figure out on their own what you are likely to emphasize. Or you may tell them that specific material will definitely be on the test so that they are certain to know something you consider very important and that another matter will definitely not need to be memorized so that studying does not become a massive rote learning experience. You may give a general guideline, such as "Material covered in the textbook and in class will be most heavily tested but you are responsible for other material in the book and from your lecture notes."

9. Are you going to use other assignments besides tests to determine grades? You might wish to adopt the philosophy that all college courses should incorporate some writing. Or perhaps you believe it is important for students to receive practice in orally presenting material. Spend some time thinking about what kinds of projects this abnormal course lends itself to easily, what students learn from different kinds of projects, and what you are interested in evaluating. In abnormal psychology, you can use fictional or non-fictional stories about a person with a mental disorder, you could assign book critiques on self-help books or more scholarly books, you can do journals, term papers, oral presentations, and so forth.

10. Will you have all students do the same type of project, or have options? How will you make the options equal (a book critique is not a term paper)? Will all students do the same number of projects (e.g., we have at times adopted the policy of requiring one project toward a C, two toward a B, and three toward an A)? Students will ask if they can do another one for extra credit, so have your answer to that ready.

11. What is your make-up test policy? Remember that commuter campuses or large numbers of non-traditional students with job and family responsibilities mean a high number of valid excuses. Can you develop a policy that is fair to students and to yourself? Our own favorite policy is to use the final exam period for multiple-choice test make-ups; students are given a chance to make up missed (or poor) tests, but those who have skipped the most tests end up punishing themselves with a comprehensive final exam—those who have been prepared throughout the semester end up being finished with the course right before the final exam period. (If you do this approach, make certain it is consistent with administrative policy. Some colleges require a mandatory final exam.)

12. What are you going to do the first day of class? Consider using this time to go through the entire syllabus explaining the "map of the course" and giving sound study tips (many college students have never been formally instructed in studying techniques). Or you might plan a dramatic, grabbing introduction to the course material.

13. If you are new on campus, check out campus resources for counseling so you can make proper and appropriate referrals if students become distressed by topics such as incest, suicide, and substance abuse.

14. Also check out the campus library and see what materials (books, journals, magazines, tapes) are available for student use. Ask the librarian how you can most appropriately utilize their services. Ask about the inter-library loan policy and policy for having reserved materials. Find out if you can influence future book purchases by the library and build materials available for your course(s).

15. Decide on your office policy (making it compatible with any school or departmental policy). Will you be available only certain hours, or can students drop by whenever you are in your office?

16. Above all, remember that you are teaching a course to which everybody can relate. All individuals have dealt with experiences of depression, anxiety, and anger. Many have been or are dealing with issues such as incest, suicide, substance abuse, and so forth. Your course has the potential to have a large influence in your students' lives. Some of the students may learn things that will help them resolve an existing problem or give them the courage to get needed treatment. Some may discover a new concern and need a direction in which to turn. Others will gain in understanding the problems of family members or friends. Others will be moved toward a career in psychology or another helping profession. Enjoy your course, but remember to take it as seriously as some of your students will take it. Be challenged by the responsibility.

Instructor Book Resources

The books listed here are only a small portion of the current resources that are available in the area of abnormal psychology and mental health treatment. I have tried to provide a list of general resources and book series and also some specific topic books. I suggest that you learn more about books in the area by attending a regional or national APA convention and collecting available booklists and by writing for materials from publishers who have several books in psychology. I advise you to peruse your campus library and also your public library to determine the quality and quantity of books already available to students. Your college librarian can suggest ways to improve the quality of resource materials in your area, such as utilizing inter-library loans and making a long-term commitment to ordering new books each year. Finally, you might want to go to local bookstores and take note of the best available self-help books.

General Reading Resources:
Adams, B.N. & Klein, D.M. (Series Eds.). *Perspectives on Marriage and the Family.* New York: Guilford. Relevant topics include social stress and family development and domestic violence.

Annual Review of Psychology. Palo Alto: Annual Reviews. Excellent material for updating in many areas of psychology.

Bellack, A.S. & Hersen, M. (Series Eds.). *Applied Clinical Psychology.* New York: Plenum. Source of material on treatment topics.

Blane, H.T. & Kosten, T.R. (Series Eds.). *The Guilford Substance Abuse Series.* New York: Guilford. Volumes include psychological theories of drinking and alcoholism, alcohol problems in women, children of alcoholics, and cocaine.

Chilman, C.S., Nunnally, E.W., & Cox, F.M. (Series Eds.). *Families in Trouble Series.* Newbury Park: Sage. Volumes include chronic illness and disability, variant family forms, and troubled relationships.

Costa, Jr., P.T., Whitfield, J. & Stewart, D. (Eds.). 1989. *Alzheimer's disease: Abstracts of the psychological and behavioral literature.* Washington, D.C.: American Psychological Association. Contains over 1180 abstracts from about 1300 journals.

Franks, V. (Series Eds.). *Springer Series: Focus on Women.* New York: Springer. A 12-volume series of major psychological and social issues on women's status and problems.

G. Stanley Hall Lecture Series. Washington, D.C.: American Psychological Association. Published annually from lectures presented at the annual APA convention. Several applicable topics.

Green, R. (Series, Ed.). *Perspectives in sexuality: Behavior, research, and therapy.* New York: Plenum. Source for material on sexual disorders.

Jones, J.L. & Kerby, J. & Landry, C.P. (Eds.). 1989. AIDS: *Abstracts of the psychological and behavioral literature, 1983-1989.* 2nd ed. Washington, D.C.: American Psychological Association. Over 650 abstracts of journal articles and 150 listings of books and chapters.

Kastenbaum, R. (Series Ed.). *Springer Series: Death and Suicide.* New York: Springer. Several volumes on death issues, with suicide and grief being especially applicable to this course.

Kazdin, A.E. (Series Ed.). *Developmental Clinical Psychology and Psychiatry Series.* Newbury Park: Sage. Topics include adolescent delinquency, chronic childhood illness, attempted suicide among youth, infant psychiatry, and child abuse.

Master Lectures. Washington, D.C.: American Psychological Association. Includes volumes on psychology and health and clinical neuropsychology and brain function.

Solnit, A.J. (Series Ed.). *The Psychoanalytic Study of the Child.* New Haven: Yale University Press. Over 40 volumes on a wide range of psychoanalytic topics.

Sonkin, D.J. (Series Ed.). *Springer Series: Focus on Men.* New York: Springer. A five-volume series of research and theoretical perspectives on topics of significance to men.

Teaching Materials and Teaching Skills:
Benjamin, Jr., L.T., Daniel, R.S. & Brewer, C.L. *Handbook for teaching introductory psychology.* Hillsdale: Lawrence Erlbaum. Selections from the first ten years of *Teaching Psychology*, including several that can be adapted to abnormal psychology courses.

Benjamin, Jr., L.T., & Lowman, K.D. (Eds.). 1988. *Activities handbook for the teaching of psychology, vol. 1.* Washington, D.C.: American Psychological Association. Contains 44 classroom activities, demonstrations, and experiments, including some for developmental psychology.

Bradley-Johnson, S. & Lesiak, J.L. 1989. *Problems in written expression: Assessment and remediation.* New York: Guilford. Provides the components essential for written communication and helps evaluate and improve deficient writing skills.

Bronstein, P. & Uina, K. 1988. *Teaching a psychology of people: Resources for gender and sociocultural awareness.* Washington, D.C.: American Psychological Association. Provides minority and cultural awareness and a variety of viewpoints, research, and experiences.

Golub, S. & Freedman, R.J. (Eds.). 1987. *Psychology of women: Resources for a core curriculum.* New York: Garland. Provides discussion topics and demonstration projects that can help developmental psychology instructors "mainstream" women's issues into their courses. Also a good source for films and book resources.

Makosky, V.P., Whitemore, L.G. & Rogers, A.M. (Eds.). *Activities handbook for the teaching of psychology, vol. 2.* Washington, D.C.: American Psychological Association. Contains about ninety activities.

McKeachie, W.J. *Teaching tips.* Lexington: D.C. Heath. Good guide for the beginning teacher.

Network: The newsletter for psychology teachers at two-year colleges. Washington, D.C.: American Psychological Association. Includes resource ideas, teaching strategies, and film reviews.

Shapiro, E.S. 1989. *Academic skills problems: Direct assessment and intervention.* New York: Guilford. Detailed instructions for evaluating and improving academic skills.

Teaching of psychology. Washington, D.C.: American Psychological Association. A quarterly journal directed toward the improvement of teaching of psychology courses. Includes course descriptions, film and book reviews, demonstrations, and useful articles.

Young, R.E. (Editor-in-chief). *New directions for teaching and learning.* San Francisco: Jossey-Bass. Published quarterly for more than a decade, these volumes give ideas and techniques for improving college teaching. Recent volumes have looked at developing critical thinking and problem-solving abilities, improving teaching styles, teaching large classes well, and teaching writing in all disciplines.

Specific Topic References:
Bagley, C. & King, K. 1989. *Child sexual abuse: The search for healing.* New York: Routledge. Overview of etiology, treatment, and prevention.

Bass, E. & Thornton, L. (Ed.). 1988. *I never told anyone: A collection of writing by survivors of child sexual abuse.* New York: Harper & Row. Collection of poetry and recollections from survivors—good to use excerpts during lectures.

Beck, A., Emery, G. & Greenberg, R. 1985. *Anxiety disorders and phobias: A cognitive perspective.* New York: Basic Books. Application of cognitive therapy to the treatment of anxiety disorders and phobias.

Beck, A., Freeman, A. et al. 1990. *Cognitive therapy of personality disorders.* New York: Guilford Press. Interesting application of cognitive therapy to each of the personality disorders.

Bemporad, J.R. & Herzog, D.B. 1989. *Psychoanalysis and eating disorders.* New York: Guilford. Looks at Freud's early views on anorexia and then reinterprets this by new developments in psychoanalysis.

Boyle, M. 1990. *Schizophrenia—A scientific delusion?.* New York: Routledge. A book that challenges schizophrenia as a disease and offers alternative explanations for bizarre behavior.

Bradburn, N.M. & Sudman, S. 1988. *Polls and surveys: Understanding what they tell us.* A guide to understanding polls and surveys. Gives material to help students understand popular polls such as Gallup, Harris, and television election night polls.

Briere, J. 1989. *Therapy for adults molested as children: Beyond survival.* New York: Springer. Topics include post-sexual abuse trauma, hysteria, borderline personality disorder, and client dissociation during therapy.

Bruch, H. 1989. *Conversations with anorexics*. New York: Basic Books. Provides material to adapt to your lectures.

Bugental, J.E.T. 1990. *Intimate journeys: Stories from life-changing therapy*. New York: Jossey-Bass. Stories of self-discovery during therapy with titles such as "I Don't Feel Fifty," "You've Been Blindfolded Since Childhood," and "Blame is All I Have Left."

Calam, R.M. & Franchi, C. 1987. *Child abuse and its consequences: Observational approaches*. New York: Cambridge University Press. Looks at long-term psychological effects of child abuse.

Crewdson, J. 1989. *By silence betrayed: Sexual abuse of children in America*. New York: Harper & Row. One of its many topics is whether pedophiles can be successfully treated.

Curran, D.K. 1987. *Adolescent suicidal behavior*. New York: Hemisphere. Provides information on many aspects of adolescent suicidal behavior.

Curtiss, S. 1977. *Genie, A psycholinguistic study of a modern-day "wild child."* New York: Academic Press. A case study of a severely neglected child who was raised without being taught language.

David, H.P. Dytrych, Z., Matejcek, Z. & Schuller, V. (Eds.). 1988. *Born unwanted: Developmental effects of denied abortion*. New York: Springer. Looks at the long-term adverse effects on children born to mothers who were refused abortions. Based on data from a study in Prague and some Scandinavian studies. Material from this book can help spark a lively class discussion.

Davis, L. 1990. *The courage to heal workbook: For women and men survivors of child sexual abuse*. Useful to show to class because some may want to buy it for personal healing.

Diamond, M. 1988. Enriching heredity: *The impact of the environment on the anatomy of the brain*. New York: Free Press. Covers three decades of research that provides evidence that at any stage of life an enriched environment can increase brain size. Useful in building lecture material on the biological aspects of mental disorders.

Diamont, L. (Ed.). *Male and female homosexuality: Psychological perspectives*. New York: Hemisphere. Includes historical approaches, ego-dystonic homosexuality, a theory of normal homosexuality, and a humanistic outlook.

Doctor, R.F. 1988. *Transvestites and transsexuals: Toward a theory of cross-gender behavior*. New York: Plenum. From fetishism through primary transsexualism, this book will provide much material for a lecture on sexual disorders.

Figley, C.R. 1989. *Helping traumatized families*. San Francisco: Jossey-Bass. A comprehensive approach to assessing and treating families experiencing stress disorders due to criminal assaults, natural disasters, and terminal illness.

Fossum, M.A. & Mason, M.J. 1989. *Facing shame: Families in recovery*. New York: Norton. Suggests that alcohol abuse, eating disorders, and child abuse may be related to an underlying process of shame.

Friedman, R.C. 1988. *Male homosexuality: A contemporary psychoanalytic perspective.* New Haven: Yale University Press. Attempts to integrate sexual orientation with psychoanalytic theory, including the role of erotic fantasy in childhood, unconscious homosexuality, and bisexuality.

Garbino, J., Guttmann, E. & Seeley, J.W. 1986. *The psychologically battered child: Strategies for identification, assessment, and intervention.* San Francisco: Jossey-Bass. Guidelines for identifying, investigating, preventing, and treating psychological maltreatment.

Gay, P. 1988. *Freud: A life for our time.* New York: Norton. You can add material about Freud's thinking and life to the introductory chapter on theoretical perspectives.

Gelles, R.J. & Cornell, C.P. 1990. *Intimate violence in families.* 2nd ed. Newbury Park, CA: Sage. Deals with contemporary attitudes, child abuse, spousal abuse, hidden victims, and society's responsibility.

Gibbs, J.T., Huang, L.N. et al. 1989. *Children of color: Psychological interventions with minority youth.* San Francisco: Jossey-Bass. A guide to assessment and treatment of minority children and adolescents, including young Blacks, Chinese, Hispanics, Japanese, Native Americans, and biracial youth.

Gournay, K. 1989. *Agoraphobia: Current perspectives on theory and treatment.* New York: Routledge. Looks at a variety of current treatments for agoraphobia patients.

Gray, J.W. & Dean, R.S. (Ed.). 1991 *Neuropsychology of perinatal complications.* New York: Springer. Deals with perinatal complications and their likely effects on later development. Deals with the importance of early intervention and the effects on education.

Green, R. 1987. *The "Sissy boy syndrome" and the development of homosexuality.* New Haven: Yale University Press. Traces the development of male homosexuality from early years into adulthood.

Heaslip, J., Van Dyke, D., Hogenson, D. & Vedders, L. 1989. *Young people and drugs: Evaluation and treatment.* Center City: Hazelden. Good for learning about the differences between evaluation and treatment of young people and that of adults.

Horton, A.L., Johnson, B.L., Roundy, L.M., & Williams, D. (Eds.). 1989. *The incest perpetrator: A family member no one wants to treat.* Newbury Park, CA: Sage. Includes a basic profile of the incest perpetrator, treatment guidelines, and referral options.

Hsu, L.K. G. 1990. *Eating disorders.* New York: Guilford. A coherent review and synthesis of the current thinking and findings on eating disorders.

Johnson, A.B. 1990. *Out of Bedlam: The truth about deinstitutionalization.* New York: Basic Books. Source of information for lectures on what happened as the hospitalization of mental patients declined by thousands.

Kagan, R. & Schlosberg, S. 1989. *Families in perpetual crisis.* New York: Norton. Information about families with long histories of chronic and severe problems.

Kernberg, O.F., Seltzer, M.A., Koenigsberg, H.W., Carr, A.C. & Appelbaum, A.H. 1989. *Psychodynamic psychotherapy of borderline patients*. New York: Basic Books. Kernberg's model of psychodynamic psychotherapy with borderline patients.

Kernberg, P.F. & Chazen, S. 1991. *Children with conduct disorders: A clinical treatment manual*. New York: Basic Books. Using individual therapy, play therapy, and parent training group therapy with treating conduct disorders in children.

Kupfer, F. 1982. *Before and after Zachariah*. New York: Delacorte. Provides a good case study of how families learn to cope with a special-needs infant.

Landau, E. 1983. *Why are they starving themselves?*. New York: Julian Messner. A guide to understanding and dealing with bulimia and anorexia nervosa.

Larsen, E. 1987. *Stage II relationships: Love beyond addiction*. San Francisco: Harper & Row. Reviews techniques for breaking unhealthy behavioral patterns that exist after attaining sobriety.

Lerman, H. 1986. *A mote in Freud's eye: From psychoanalysis to the psychology of women*. New York: Springer. Examines Freud's attitudes toward women and how that influenced his theory. Also traces Freud's influences to present-day psychoanalytic theories. Useful for enriching class discussions on psychoanalytic theory.

Lifton, R.J. & Markusen, E. 1990. *The genocidal mentality: Nazi holocaust and nuclear threat*. New York: Basic Books. Looks at the forces behind the rise of the genocidal mentality.

Marlin, E. 1987. *Hope: New choices and recovery strategies for adult children of alcoholics*. How ACOAs can attain emotional health.

Marlin, E. 1990. *Relationships in recovery: Healing strategies for couples and families*. New York: Harper & Row. Relationships between codependents and alcoholics and how to make them healthier.

Mellody, P., Miller, A.W., & Miller, J.K. 1989. *Facing co-dependence*. San Francisco: Harper & Row. Traces the beginnings of co-dependent patterns back to childhood.

Miller, N. 1990. *In search of gay America*. New York: Harper & Row. Add to historical and contemporary lecture information on homosexuality.

Nelkin, D. & Tancredi, L. 1989. *Dangerous diagnostics: The social power of biological information*. New York: Basic Books. Uses and possible misuses of biological tests, like DNA mapping and PET scans in work, court, and school settings.

Newcomb, M.D. & Bentler, P.M. 1988. *Consequences of adolescent drug use: Impact on the lives of young adults*. Newbury Park: Sage. Looks at the effects of adolescent drug use on deviant behavior, sexual behavior, mental health, and family issues.

164

Orbach, I. 1988. *Children who don't want to live: Understanding and treating the suicidal child.* San Francisco: Jossey-Bass. Compares adult suicides and child suicides. Explores children's attempts, threats, and messages as well as looking at personality and life circumstances factors.

Rosenthal, D. 1963. *The Genain quadruplets.* New York: Basic Books. Source of lecture material for relating about a set of quadruplets all diagnosed as schizophrenic.

Steinmetz, S.K. 1988. *Duty bound: Elder abuse and family care.* Newbury Park, CA: Sage. Looks at abuse toward the elderly by their family caretakers.

Sweeney, T.J. 1989. *Adlerian counseling: A practical approach for a new decade.* 3rd ed. Muncie: Accelerated Development. Includes major life tasks, interrelatedness of early recollections and present behavior, and usefulness in therapy. Many of Adler's concepts fit well into an undergraduate abnormal psychology course.

Taylor, R.L. 1990. *Distinguishing psychological from organic disorders: Screening for psychological masquerade.* New York: Springer. An informative, readable book that informs one how to distinguish medical conditions from psychological problems. Especially good at providing interesting case studies, including one on George Gershwin.

Valenstein, E.S. 1987. *Great and desperate cures: The rise and decline of psychosurgery and other radical treatments for mental illness.* New York: Basic Books. An interesting definitive history of lobotomy that can provide interesting quotes and statistics for class lectures.

Virtue, D.L. 1989. *The yo-yo syndrome diet.* New York: Harper & Row. The pattern of losing the same ten to fifty pounds over and over during one's lifetime.

Washton, A. & Boundy, D. 1988. *Willpower's not enough: Understanding and overcoming addiction and obsessive behavior.* New York: Harper & Row. Provides the same formula for gamblers, workaholics, and drug abusers. Belief that patterns of dependence arise from the addict's own personality.

Washton, A. 1989. *Cocaine addiction: Treatment, recovery, and relapse prevention.* New York: Norton. Clinical assessment and treatment of cocaine and crack addiction.

Weinrech, J.D. 1987. *Sexual landscapes: Why we are what we are, why we love whom we love.* New York: Charles Scribner's Sons. Explores sociobiology of sex, core gender identity, and sexual orientation.

Westkott, M. 1986. *The feminist legacy of Karen Horney.* New Haven: Yale University Press. Looks at Karen Horney's theory and its central theme of women's conflict between dependency and ambition. Can tie into many modern topics, including co-dependency and stress from balancing career, marriage, and parenthood.

White, G.L. & Mullen, P.E. 1989. *Jealousy: Theory, research, and clinical strategies.* New York: Guilford. Deals with both normal and pathological romantic jealousies.

Windle, M. & Searles, J.S. (Eds.). 1990. *Children of alcoholics: Critical perspectives*. New York: Guilford. A wide range of topics and a critical evaluation of COA research.

Wolff, L. 1988. *Postcards from the end of the world: Child abuse in Freud's Vienna*. New York: Atheneum. Can be used to elaborate how Freud's zeitgeist influenced his theoretical ideas or to give a historical perspective to your lecture on child abuse.

Wyatt, G.E. & Powell, G.J. 1988. *Lasting effects of child sexual abuse*. Newbury Park: Sage. The lasting effects of child sexual abuse upon child victims, adult survivors, and their families.

General Resources: Film and Videotape List

One of the first tasks you should do in developing your abnormal psychology course is to make decisions about which media to use and when. It is usually necessary to reserve your media choices even before the semester begins, especially if you want to utilize the media on a specific class period. You should first check with your college's media department/library to (1) learn their procedures for booking materials; (2) see if the college owns any media on abnormal psychology topics, (3) learn of any budget constraints on your choices, and (4) find out if they have a collection of media resource catalogs that you can peruse. You might want to begin a collection of media catalogs and you can do this by requesting catalogs from the film distributors listed at the end of this section or by picking up catalogues from film distributors with a display at regional or national APA conventions. These conventions also provide screenings of the newest media choices so that you can make good decisions about which items are most appropriate. Some media choices are provided here on some general and popular topics in psychology.

Theoretical Positions:

Being Abraham Maslow (FML, 30 min., b&w). Autobiography of Abraham Maslow, including Maslow talking about his childhood, education, professional conflicts, and overall philosophy (film, video).

B.F. Skinner and Behavior Change: Research, Practice, and Promise (RP, 45 min.). Behavioral interventions in various settings, including fear of dental procedures, learning social skills at a youth center, controlling epilepsy in a hospital, and working with a developmentally disabled child at home (film, video).

C.G. Jung: A Matter of Heart (IM, 107 min.). Jung's biography (video).

Everybody Rides the Carousel (YU, 24 min., 1982). A presentation of Erikson's theory of human life cycle (film).

Freud Under Analysis (MINN, 58 min., 1987). Deals with Freud's beliefs and the scientific evidence (video).

The Humanistic Revolution: Pioneers in Perspective (PEF, 32 min., b&w). Interviews with Maslow, Murphy, Rogers, May, Tillich, Perls, Frankl, and Watts (film, video).

In Search of the Soul (MINN, 30 min., 1972). Jung's childhood years and his years with Freud (video).

Observational Learning (H&R, 23 min., 1978). Introduction to the social learning approach with examples of the effects of parents, peers, and the media (film).

Rollo May on Humanistic Psychology (PEF, 24 min.). May describes the historical development and general characteristics of humanistic psychology (film, video).

Models of Abnormality:
Keltie's Beard: A Woman's Story (FML, 9 min., 1983). A woman with heavy facial hair that she does not bother to cut. Useful in discussing the criteria for abnormal (film, video).

Little People (FML, 58 min., 1985). The discrimination and difficulties of access for dwarfs. Good for discussing definition and meaning of abnormal (film, video).

Mental Retardation/Organic Brain Syndrome/Learning Disabilities:
Autistic Child: A Behavioral Approach (MINN, 26 min., 1982). Describes symptoms and etiology of autism. Looks at behavioral treatments (film).

Backwards: The Riddle of Dyslexia (SSC, 30 min., 1985). Explains learning disabilities and treatment (film).

Grandma Didn't Wave Back (FHS, 24 min.). A family dealing with senility due to Alzheimer's (film, video).

Learning Disabilities (FHS, 19 min.). Case study of a 9-year-old revealing symptoms, diagnosis, and treatment (video).

Learning Disability: A Family Crisis (MVP, 41 min., 1989). A family deals with an 8-year-old just diagnosed as having a learning disability (video).

May's Miracle: A Retarded Youth with a Gift for Music (FML, 28 min., 1983). A blind, retarded, cerebral palsied "idiot savant" who is musically talented (video).

Substance Abuse:
Addiction and the Family (FHS, 19 min.). Family's role in recovery (video).

Continued Acts of Sabotage (HAZ, 35 min., 1989). Five individuals and their erratic pathways toward recovery (film, video).

Crack (FHS, 28 min.). The warning signs of crack use, long-term consequences, treatment (video).

Crack Street, USA: First Person Experiences (IM, 29 min., 1989). Ex-users address the devastating effects of crack (video).

Crystal (FHS, 56 min). Documentary about crystal and its effects on users (video).

Designer Drugs (FHS, 28 min.). Synthetic drugs and possible permanent brain damage (video).

A Family Talks about Alcohol (PER, 25 min.). The physiological effects of alcohol and how family members deal with an alcoholic (film).

From Use to Abuse (HAZ). Looks at how chemical use becomes substance abuse.

Growing Up in Smoke (MTI, 15 min., 1984). Messages to young people about cigarette use and contrasts industry's and health officials' positions on the effects of smoking (film).

Smoking/Emphysema: A Fight for Breath (CRM, 12 min). The difference in healthy vs. diseased lungs (film, video).

Sons and Daughters/Drugs and Booze (RG, 28 min.). Provides practical advice and information to parents and their children who use alcohol and drugs (film).

168

Staying Sober, Keeping Straight (HAZ, 35 min, 1989). Scenarios follow recovering individuals confronted with common relapse triggers (film, video).

Steroids and Sports (FHS, 19 min.). Use of steroids to increase performance and increased physical risks (video).

Targets (MINN, 19 min., 1985). After an alcohol-related accident, teens make insight into dealing with personal problems (film).

Viable Alternatives (HAZ). Alternatives to chemical use and abuse.

Eating Disorders:
Anorexia and Bulimia (FHS, 19 min). The addictive nature of eating disorders and the biological damage (video).

Bulimia (CRM, 12 min., 1983). Describes bulimia and the motives of its victims (film).

Bulimia: The Binge-Purge Obsession (RP, 20 min.). The causes and effects of bulimia among high school and college students (film, video).

Less than Nothing: Anorexia (IM). Case study of a female adolescent with anorexia (video).

Portraits of Anorexia (MINN, 28 min., 1987). Seven anorexics are interviewed and address their expectations, behaviors, and relationships (video).

The Waist Land: Eating Disorders (MINN, 23 min., 1985). Obsession with thinness and the resulting eating disorders (video).

You Can Be Too Thin: Understanding Anorexia and Bulimia (IM). A case study of one female's eating disorder and treatment (video).

Sexuality and Sexual Disorders:
Homosexuality: Nature vs. Nurture (FHS, 26 min.). Biological, genetic, psychological, and cultural explanations of sexual orientation (video).

Homosexuality: "What about McBride?" (CRM, 10 min., 1975). Two friends argue over whether to include a third boy on a raft trip when the third boy is thought to be a homosexual (film).

Michael, A Gay Son (FML, 27 min., 1981). Michael "comes out" and deals with peer reactions and parental rejection (film).

Sexual Addiction (HAZ, 45 min., 1989). Defines sexual addiction and explores similarities to chemical dependency and its treatment (video).

169

Abuse: Emotional, Physical, Verbal, Sexual:

ACA Recovery: Meeting the Child Within (MINN, 25 min., 1989). Adult recovery from childhood realities of alcoholic families (video).

Adult Children of Alcoholics (MINN, 30 min., 1988). Understanding their problems and typical behaviors (video).

Adult Children of Alcoholics: The Masks of Denial (MINN, 23 min., 1987). The psychological/emotional problems of dealing up with an alcoholic parent (film).

Babies Are People Too (CF, 27 min., 1985). An anti-infant abuse film (film).

Battered Teens (FI, 16 min., 1982). Battered and neglected adolescents (film).

The Battering Syndrome (IM, 45 min.). Battered spouses and children, typical triggering phenomenon, assistance (video).

Children in Peril (IM, 22 min.). A tour of several agencies and hospitals where battered children are treated (video).

Child Abuse: Breaking the Cycle (IM). Three individuals tell their stories about being abused/abusers (video).

Generations of Violence (FML, 55 min., 1989). How abused children sometimes grow up to become abusive parents and possible solutions (video).

Incest, the Family Secret (FML, 57 min., 1984). Women's stories of being traumatized in their youth by incestuous fathers, lack of protection by mothers, and treatment of one abusive father (video).

Men Who Molest: Children Who Survive (FML, 52 min., 1985). Four child molesters and their treatment; child victims, their families, and their treatment (film, video).

The Unquiet Death of Eli Creekmore (FML, 55 min., 1988). A documentary of a brutal child abuse case in which a preschooler is beaten to death for crying at the dinner table (video).

Trust in Yourself: Adult Children of Alcoholics (MINN, 25 min., 1988). Deals with the power of denial and confusion, and the healing potential of forgiveness and group therapy (video).

Suicide:

Adolescent Suicide: A Matter of Life and Death (APGA, 39 min., 1983). Teenage suicide problem (film).

Childhood's End: A Look at Adolescent Suicide (FML, 28 min., 1981). The emotional and complex issues around adolescent suicide (film, video).

Dead Serious (MTI, 24 min., 1987). Major factors contributing to teenage suicide (film, video).

Everything to Live for (FHS, 52 min.). Features two attempted suicides and two completed suicides among teens and their survivors (video).

Gifted Adolescents and Suicide (FHS, 26 min.). The suicide risks of super-achiever teens (video).

Sometimes I Wonder If It's Worth It (AIT, 30 min., 1986). Three teen survivors of suicide attempts and parents of one who died tell their stories (video).

Suicide: Teenage Crisis (CRM, 10 min., 1981). Suicide's prevalence and possible solutions (film).

Media Distributor Addresses:

ABC	ABC Merchandising, 330 W. 42nd St., New York, NY 10036
ABCNC	ABC News Closeup, 157 Columbus Avenue, 4th Floor, New York, NY 10023
BCN	Beacon Films, P.O. Box 575, 1250 Washington St., Norwood, MA 02062
BF	Benchmark Films, Inc. 145 Scarborough Road, Briarcliff Manor, NY 10510
CDF	Cambridge Documentary Films, P.O. Box 385, Cambridge, MA 02139
CFV	Carousel Film & Videos, 241 E. 34th St., Room 304, New York, NY 10167
CBS	CBS Enterprises, 245 Park Avenue, 34th Floor, New York, NY 10167
CP	Centre Productions, Inc., 1800 30th St., Room 304, New York, NY 10167
CM	Concept Media, P.O. Box 19542, Irvine, CA 92714
CG	Cinema Guild, 1697 Broadway, Room 802, New York, NY 10019
CRM	CRM/McGraw-Hill Films, 110 15th St., Del Mar, CA 92014
DAV	Davidson Films, 3701 Buchanan St., San Francisco, CA 94123
DP	Dean Productions, Josephine, 205 W. End Ave., New York, NY 10023
ECC	Educational Cable Consortium, 24 Beechwood Road, Summit, NJ 07901
EDC	Educational Development Center, Distrib. Ctr., 39 Chapel St., Newton, MA 02160
FI	Films, Inc., 5547 Ravenswood Ave., Chicago, IL 60640
FML	Filmmakers Library, Inc., 133 E. 58th St., Ste. 703A, New York, NY 10022
GA	Guidance Associates, 757 3rd Ave., New York, NY 10017
HBJ	Harcourt Brace Jovanovich, 757 3rd Ave., New York, NY 10017
H&R	Harper & Row Media, 10 E. 53rd St., New York, NY 10022
HRM	Human Relations Media, 175 Tompkins Ave., Pleasantville, NY 10570
IM	Insight Media, 121 W. 85th St., New York, NY 10024
JBL	J.B. Lippincott Co., E. Washington Square, Philadelphia, PA 19105
KSU	Kent State University, Audio Visual Services, Kent, OH 44242
LMP	Larry Madison Productions, 111 E. 39th St., New York, NY 10016
LCA	Learning Corp. of America, 108 Wilmot Road, Deerfield, IL 60015
MF	Milner-Fenwick, Inc. 3800 Liberty Heights Ave., Baltimore, MD 21215
MM	Motavision Media, 2 Parktree Court, Chico, CA 95926
MTI	MTI Teleprograms, 3710 Commercial Ave., Northbrook, IL 60062
NFBC	Nat'l Film Board of Canada, 1251 Avenue of the Americas, New York, NY 10036
NYU	New York University Film Library, 26 Washington Place, New York, NY 10013
NLP	Northern Lights Productions, 165 Newbury St., Boston, MA 02116
PBS	Public Broadcasting System, 1320 Braddock Place, Alexandria, VA 22314
PER	Perennial Education, Inc., 1825 Willow Road, Northfield, IL 60091
PF	Pyramid Films, P.O. Box 1048, Santa Monica, CA 90406
PFV	Phoenix Films & Videos, 470 Park Ave. South, New York, NY 10016
PMF	Parents Magazine Films, Inc., 52 Vanderbilt Ave., New York, NY 10017
POLY	Polymorph Films, Inc., 118 South St., Boston, MA 02115
RP	Research Press, Box 31772, Champaign, IL 61820
SBC,SC	Sunburst Communications, 39 Washington Ave., Pleasantville, NY 10570; P.O. Box 9542, Irvine, CA 92714
SP	Sterling Productions, Ste 916, 500 N. Dearborn St., Chicago, IL 60610
SSC	Simon and Schuster Comm., Tollway North, 108 Wilmot, Deerfield, IL 60015
T-L	Time-Life Films, 43 W. 16th St., New York, NY 10011
WK	Walter J. Klein Co., Ltd., 6301 Carmel Rd., P.O. Box 220766, Charlotte, NC 28222
YWP	York/Wiley Productions, Inc., 605 3rd Ave., New York, NY 10016